DR. SEBI
MEAL PREP
COOKBOOK

1000 Day Quick & Easy Meals for the Busy. With Meal Plans and Shopping Lists

By

KERRI M. WILLIAMS

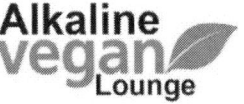

Alkaline vegan Lounge

www.alkalineveganlounge.com

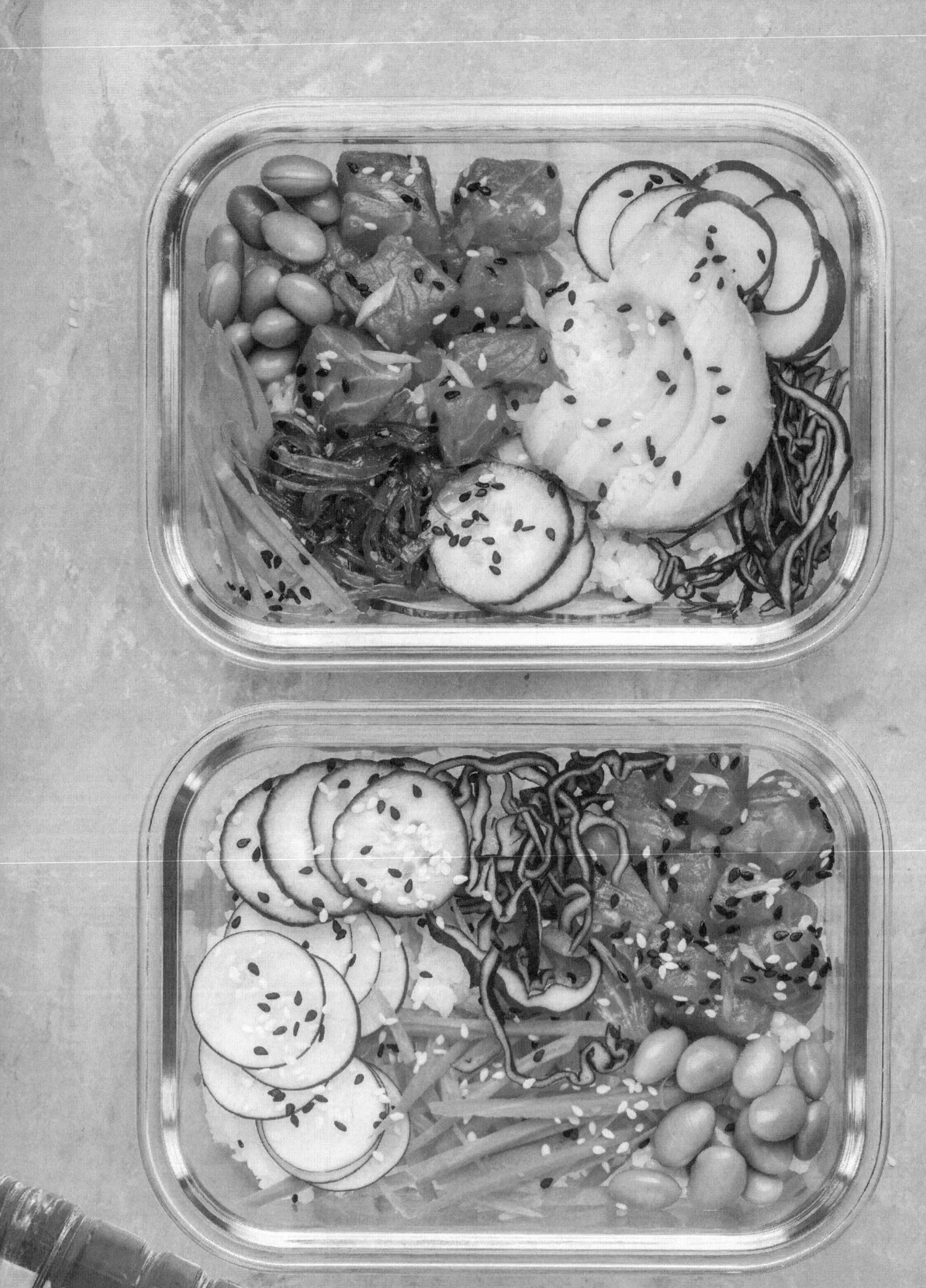

Contents

JOIN OUR COMMUNITY

Join our community of growing enthusiasts committed to the lifestyle. Also, we occasionally run discount promos for our books and other resources, and you'd be pleased to sign up to our exclusive list to get access for free. It's an amazing and growing community where we share tips and resources to help in our journey towards healthy living. Copy the link below and paste in your browser to join for free

https://manage.kmail-lists.com/subscriptions/subscribe?a=X7eqXQ&g=YdcvB2

FREE SEBI DIET STARTER KIT

Download our free Dr. Sebi Diet starter kit where you are furnished with step by step plan on how to get started on the Alkaline vegan diet. Copy the link below and paste in your browser to download your free 12-page Dr. Sebi Diet starter kit booklet now

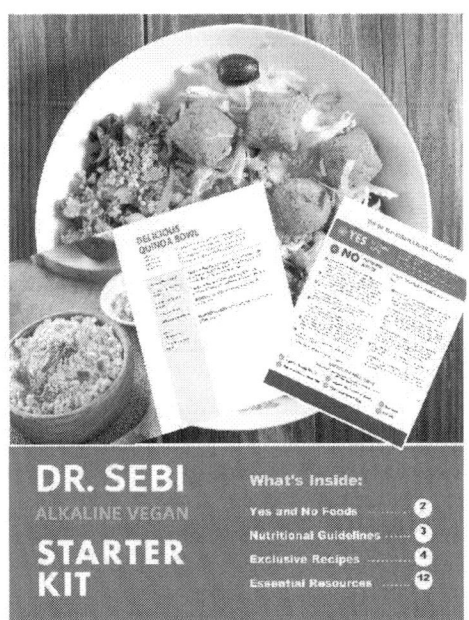

https://manage.kmail-lists.com/subscriptions/subscribe?a=X7eqXQ&g=QQnWdy

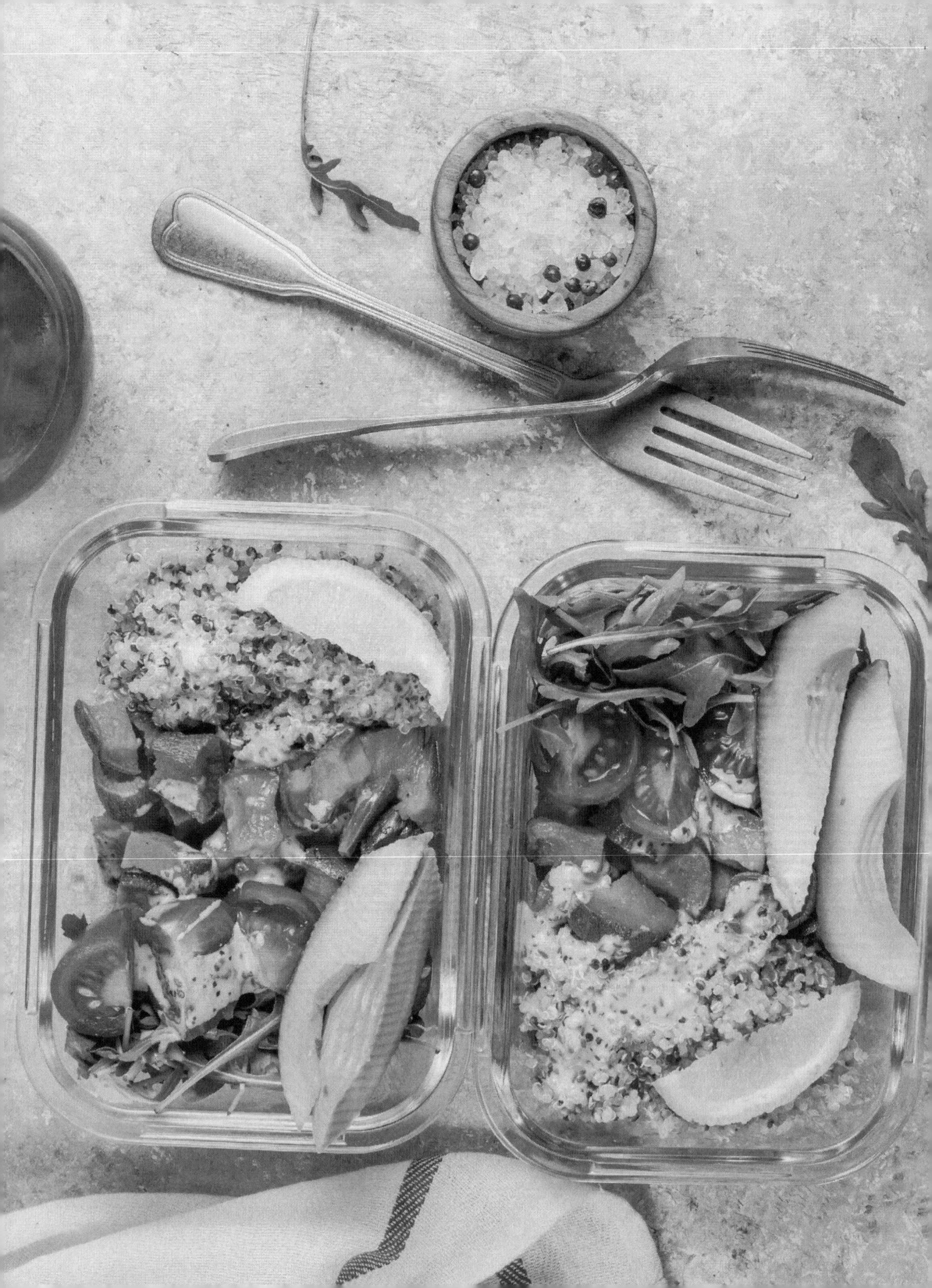

Introduction

The Alkaline Vegan Meal Prep

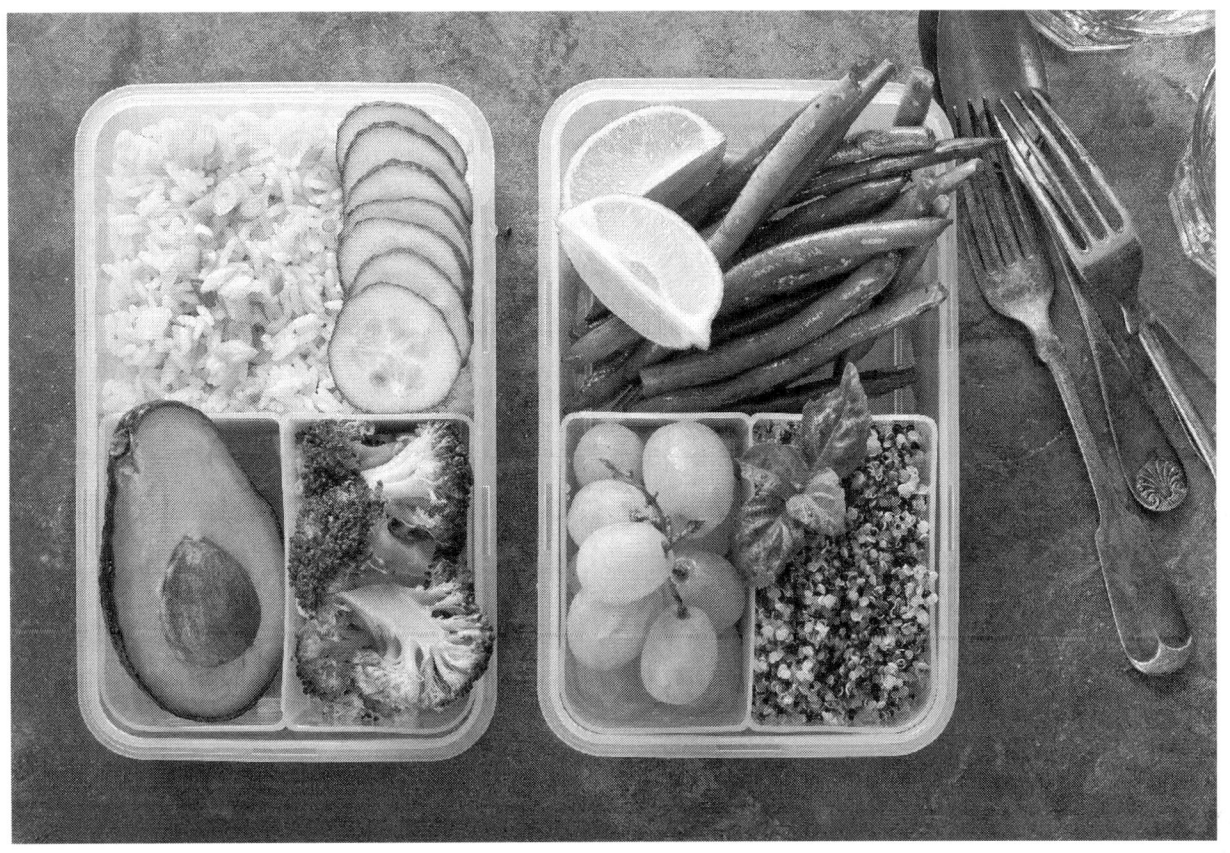

Why Choose Meal Prep?

To cope with change, you have to be ready to change. The increasingly busy lifestyle has made many people take a more critical look at their daily habits and forced them to adapt to changed circumstances. Many employed people are away from home for most of the day, which leaves very little time for cooking. This is why they either eat out, order take-aways, or eat convenient foods that are usually unhealthy. Fortunately, there is a way of following a healthy diet without having to spend hours in the kitchen every day. The secret called meal prepping has improved the eating habits of millions of people worldwide.

What is Meal Prepping?

Meal prepping is about living in an organized fashion and planning and preparing your meals ahead of time. As an idea, meal prepping is ideal for those with a hectic schedule, a large family, or someone who works long hours and gets home late too tired to cook from scratch. In other words, for all those who do not have a lot of time on their hands or who for other reasons can't, or don't want to, cook every day.

Successful meal prepping requires a strategic approach. Thinking this through may take some time but this pays in the long-term.

5 steps for meal prepping:

1. Having a plan
2. Making a shopping list
3. Shopping
4. Preparing
5. Storing

Although this may sound like a lot of work, once this becomes a routine, you'll realize how much time and money you can save this way. The reason many people don't want to try meal prepping is that they believe that this would waste what little free time they have available. However, it's more likely that many people dislike or can't afford an organized life. They eat when they have time and what they happen to lay their hands on. Take-outs have become a way of life for many simply because many people can't be bothered to plan their lives, let alone their meals. However, for those that would like more stability and order in their life, meal prepping is definitely something they would enjoy and would benefit from. There are different approaches to meal prepping so depending on your circumstances and preferences, you can choose the one that suits you most.

3 ways of organizing meal prepping:

1. Make-ahead meals

This is about preparing and cooking meals in advance and keeping them in a fridge or freezer until required. All you have to do is reheat them.

2. Batch cooking

With this method, you prepare a large quantity of a specific recipe, divide it into several smaller portions, and keep it a freezer.

3. Ready-to-cook ingredients

Another option is to prepare ingredients that will be required for the meals you plan to cook at a later stage and freeze them. For example, you can peel and chop vegetables, grate apples, squeeze juice, etc. Then, when you decide to cook something, all you need to do is combine the right ingredients and your meal will be ready in less than half an hour. However, make sure not to mix fresh and frozen veggies as some of the veggies will be overcooked and others undercooked.

We all have different lifestyles and responsibilities so depending on how early you have to leave in the morning, how late you come home in the evening, how many people you have to cook for, how much you enjoy preparing food, etc. you should choose a method that suits you most.

If planning and cooking ahead for a whole week seems like too much work, try meal prepping for just 2-3 days. If it goes well and you realize this helps you save time, you may start cooking for a couple of weeks ahead. Meal prepping for a big family or for family members with different dietary requirements does complicate things a bit but what you can do in that case is to prepare only one meal, ie the main meal, rather than meal prep for breakfast, lunch, and dinner for all family members.

Meal Prepping Benefits

Besides helping you live a more organized life; meal prepping comes with additional benefits.

4 key benefits of meal prepping:

1. You save money
When you cook ahead, you usually cook a large quantity of food which means you buy ingredients in bulk. Buying in bulk is one of the ways of cutting down on your food costs.

2. You save time
Our lives have become very busy so even those who enjoy cooking and don't mind spending a few hours in the kitchen every day, often find it hard to live this way. And if you never enjoyed cooking and cook only when you have to, meal prepping is definitely something you should consider.

3. You stick to the Dr. Sebi Diet plan

Some diets require special foods and if you happen to run out of those foods, you will probably eat whatever is available, e.g. foods that are not allowed on Dr. Sebi Food list. On the other hand, if you plan your meals ahead, and shop accordingly, you will always have the ingredients you need for Dr. Sebi-approved meals.

4. You eat healthier

Statistics show that when you plan your meals, you are much more likely to eat healthy than when you prepare a meal from what you happen to find in your fridge. For example, on Dr. Sebi Alkaline diet you know exactly what foods you should never eat so, in order not to be tempted, you will not buy such foods and will keep only the foods that are allowed on this diet.

Chapter 1

Alkaline Meal Prep Basics

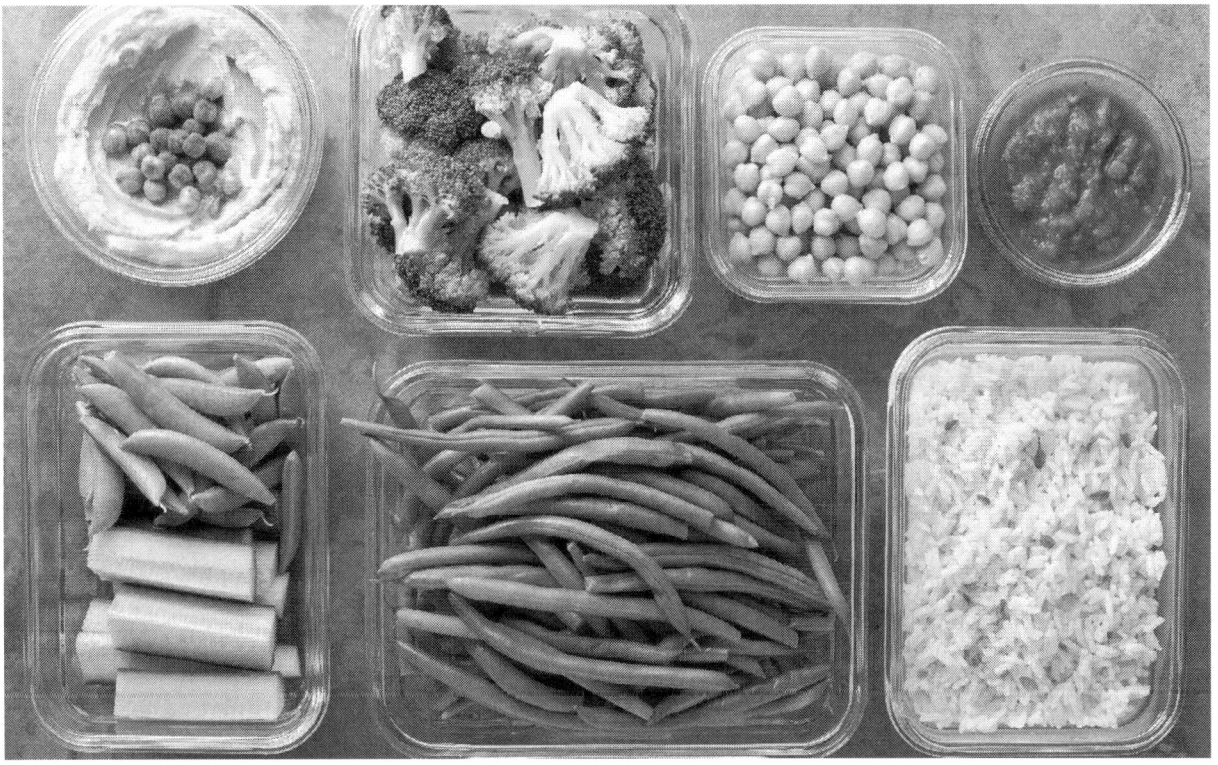

The meal prep basics revolve around preparing meals ahead of time and storing them in a way that will preserve their nutrients, flavor, and color. To achieve this, certain rules need to be followed.

Containers

Healthy food stored in the wrong way or wrong containers is a waste of time and money. As meal prepping is cooking for a few days or weeks, ahead, such meals are usually frozen or kept in the fridge. Either way, you need containers to keep the food in. Many different types of containers are available today and they come with different advantages, storing capacities, and prices. As proper storage can affect how a meal keeps and how it tastes, it's very important to choose containers that will help improve the taste rather than ruin it. But, before you go shopping for containers, make sure you know what you're going to use them for, e.g. for reheating, deep-freezing, pantry storage, etc.

<u>11 common types of containers:</u>

1. Grab-and-Go containers
2. Glass containers
3. Stainless steel containers
4. BPA-free containers
5. Stackable containers
6. Leakproof containers
7. Dishwasher-safe/Oven-safe containers
8. Microwave-safe containers
9. Freezer-safe containers
10.   Compartmentalized containers
11.   Airtight containers

Other things to consider when choosing containers is if you need reusable or single-use ones. Besides, containers are made from different materials which range from simple food plastic bags to sturdy ones made of plastic, silicone or stainless steel. However, most containers are made of plastic and if you are environmentally conscious, you can get some eco-friendly ones made from stainless steel, glass or bamboo. Personally, I like to go for over-safe glass containers. Although, they are pricey, the value you get from the investment is worth every penny. Another thing to consider is the shape and size. If you plan to store a huge amount of food or if you have very little freezing space, stackable containers would probably be the best. Alternatively, get some simple plastic food bags.

Basic Food Storage Guidelines

How tasty and healthy your frozen meals will depend not only on the ingredients used and your cooking methods but also on the way they were stored. Proper storage helps your meals retain as much of their natural flavor and nutrients as possible. So, knowing how to prepare meals is only half the job. They also need to be stored, frozen, defrosted, and reheated correctly. How long foods can be kept in a fridge or a freezer before their nutrients are affected, depends of the type of food but also on how they were processed. However, even deep-frozen foods cannot stay frozen indefinitely.

Alkaline Vegan Cold Food Storage Chart

Produce	Optimal storage temp (F)	Optimal storage temp C	Storage Life
Apples	30-40	-1 -4	1-12 months
Avocado, ripe	38-45	+3 - +7	
Avocado, unripe	45-50	+7 - +10	
Burro bananas, green	62-70	17 – 21	
Burro bananas, ripe	56-60	13 – 16	
Basil	52-59	11 – 15	
Beans, dry	40-50		6 – 10 months
Beans, green	40-45		7 – 10 days
Blackberries	32-33	0 – 1	2-3 days
Blueberries	32-35	0 – 2	
Cantaloupe	36-38	2 – 3	
Cherries, sour	32	0	3 – 7 days
Cherries, sweet	32	0	2 – 3 weeks
Cucumber	50-55		10 - 14 days
Currants	31-32		1-4 weeks
Lettuce	32	0	2-3 weeks
Figs	32-35	0 – 2	
Herbs	32-35	0 – 2	
Kale	32		2 – 3 weeks
Limes	48-55	9 – 13	
Mango	50-55	10 – 13	
Mushrooms	32	0	3 – 4 days
Peaches	31-32		2 – 4 weeks

Pears	29-31		2 – 7 months
Plums	31-32		2 – 5 weeks
Prunes	31-32		2 – 5 weeks
Squash	41-50		1 – 2 weeks
Strawberries	32	0	3 – 7 days
Turnip greens	32		10 – 14 days
Watercress	32		2 – 3 weeks
Tomatillo	55-70		4 – 7 days

Cold Food Storage Chart

Food	Type	Fridge (40ºF or 5ºC, or below)	Freezer (0 deg F or -18 C or below)
Soups & Stews		3-5 days	2-3 months
Leftovers	Cooked food, patties Pizza	3-4 days 3-4 days 3-4 days	2-6 months 1-3 months 1-2 months

Must-Have Kitchen Equipment for Sebian Meal Prep

Most activities require certain tools and this also applies to cooking. Must-have kitchen equipment can be categorized according to its purpose.

<u>5 types of kitchen equipment:</u>

1. Cutlery

These are spoons, knives, forks, ladle, spatula, tongs, slotted spoon, whisk, etc.

2. Slicing tools

Anything used for cutting, chopping, mashing or grinding falls into this category - knives, grater, potato masher, vegetable peeler, etc.

3. Oven-safe storage containers

There's nothing as convenient as taking your meal prep containers out of the refrigerator and right into the oven. Try storing your prepped foods in different containers if they will require different methods of reheating. For example, my quinoa would go straight to the steamer.

4. A Crock-pot

A great tool for lunch or reheating prepped meals.

5. A Powerful Blender

6. A Food Processor of Juicer

7. A Toaster Oven

8. A Tea Kettle

9. Pans and Pots

10.   Special extras (optional)

These can help but you can easily do without them, e.g. spiralizer, an instant pot, air fryer, a tool for zesting key limes, steamer basket, sandwich maker, immersion blender, etc.

11.   Miscellaneous

These are uncategorized items found in most kitchens, e.g. can opener, corkscrew, measuring cups or spoons, pepper mill, salad spinner, colander/strainer, cutting board, pots and pans, mixing bowls, etc.

Some of these tools are essential and no kitchen should be without them, e.g. cutlery, pots and pans, etc. Others, you should get if you can but there is no need to try and get them all at the same time. You can start by getting one or a couple from each of the categories and gradually add new ones if you think you need them. However, if you can't get most of these tools don't fret, our grandmothers prepared fantastic meals although they had very few pieces of cooking equipment and often did not even have electricity. Besides, what tools you'll need in your kitchen depends not only on your budget but also on the type of meals you are likely to prepare. For example, if smoothies are part of your diet, you will need a blender, if you bake often you will need kitchen scales, etc.

Freeze Storage Tips

If you can't cook with fresh ingredients, dry or frozen ones will do. They are not ideal but are definitely healthier than the canned ones. If frozen properly, vegetables retain most of their nutrients, flavor, and color. The trick with cooking with frozen vegetables is to prepare them in a way to make them taste as much as fresh ones as possible.

3 main rules when cooking with frozen veggies:

- Don't mix them with fresh ones because they require different cooking time;
- Don't thaw frozen veggies before cooking as they usually contain a lot of water (although there are exceptions to this rule);
- Use frozen vegetables within 10 months from freezing or within 24 hours from defrosting;

However, although freezer storage is very convenient and can help you eat fruits and vegetables throughout the year or buy and store food when it's cheap (e.g. when certain fruits or vegetables are in season), the food needs to be frozen in a way that will make its shelf life longer and identification easier.

6 tips for correct freezer storage:

1. Maintain adequate temperature

Make sure the temperature of your freezer remains consistent otherwise the food may continuously thaw and refreeze. When this happens, crystals will form on the surface of the frozen foods (i.e. freezer burn) and their nutrients will be depleted. Besides, make sure the door seals properly and keep the temperature at 0 degrees Fahrenheit (or -18 degrees C) or lower.

2. Cool thoroughly

Cool the food you plan to freeze thoroughly before putting in the fridge or freezer otherwise it will raise the temperature.

3. Keep the food in containers with lids on

Whatever type of container you use, make sure it's sealed (if it's a plastic food bag) or tightly closed with a lid. When frozen food is exposed to the air you end up with freezer burn and it loses both the flavor (especially fruits) and the nutrients.

4. Make a list of stored foods or label the containers

If you have a big freezer or keep a lot of frozen food, make sure all containers are labeled and dated. This is not necessary only in the case of original packages.

5. Keep the freezer tidy

Try to keep your freezer tidy and use different drawers to store different types of foods, e.g. fruits, veggies, soups, baked goods, leftovers, etc. If you don't have freezer drawers, you can use big plastic boxes to store specific items.

6. Avoid overcrowding

A freezer that has too many items inside is likely not to freeze well or to take much longer to achieve the desired temperature once you add more food inside. When your freezer becomes overcrowded it's a sign it's time to start using some of the foods or to stop adding new items.

Foods That Do Not Freeze Well

Although most foods can be frozen, some change their texture and appearance so much, they become inedible.

14 foods you should never try to freeze:

1. Cream-based soups and sauces
2. Cucumber
3. Desserts
4. Frostings
5. Fried foods (become soggy)
6. Fully cooked pasta (can be frozen in dishes if undercooked)
7. Fully cooked rice
8. Gelatin
9. Lettuce

The moisture content of foods changes during freezing. Ideally, it should remain within the 2-3% variance of the original state.

5 tips on freezing:

1. The optimal freezing temperature is 0 degrees F or -18 degrees C.

2. No food should be kept if a freezer for more than 6 months.

3. Big chunks of vegetable, bread or other foods should be broken down into portion sizes and individually wrapped in plastic. Keep them in

resealable freezer bags and try to remove as much air as possible.

4. Label and date all products before freezing especially if you have a big freezer or keep a lot of frozen food.

5. Maximize air circulation around fresh foods by placing it on a wire rack.

Thawing Tips

Different foods require different thawing time. You need to be particularly careful with perishable foods. These should never be thawed in hot water or left at room temperature for more than two hours.

2 common methods of food thawing:

1. Refrigerator Thawing

Big chunks of foods may require as long as 24 hours to be thawed. However, even smaller pieces of food may require a whole day. Once defrosted, most may remain in the fridge for a couple of days before cooking. Never freeze food after it's been thawed. Although it may be perfectly safe to use, it will definitely have lost a lot of its nutrients as well as flavor.

2. Coldwater thawing

If you need to thaw food quickly, you can try keeping it in cold water, provided it's been stored in leakproof containers. That will ensure it remains free of bacteria and retains its flavor. The water must not be hot and this method may take about 4 hours. You should use cold water and change it every 30 minutes. Small packages of food may thaw in less than an hour. However, should you decide to freeze this food again, it must first be cooked.

Reheating Tips

To avoid poisoning, thawed food should be reheated only once. What you haven't used, should be discarded.

Successful reheating tips:

- Ideally, you should use all the leftovers kept in the fridge within three days.

- If using leftovers from a freezer, use them within 24 hours. Defrost them thoroughly before reheating. You can do this by leaving them in the fridge for a day or popping them in the oven.
- Reheat food by making it very hot. Simmer on low heat and stir it through to make sure it's heated throughout.
- Don't reheat food more than once. The more times you cool and reheat food, the higher the risk of food poisoning. Bacteria multiplies easily when reheated food is insufficiently hot.
- Reheating rice is particularly tricky. Rice that has been cooked should not be used however if you do use it, make sure it's reheated properly until it's piping hot before serving. This can be done by simmering on low heat for a couple more minutes. This is necessary because cooked rice may contain certain types of bacteria that are resistant to heat.

10 Tips on Going Microwave-Free

The Healthiest Ways to Reheat Food

1. Steam foods that tend to get sticky, especially grains like rice or pasta
2. Simmer with a little liquid to prevent burning. You can use a few ounces of oil or just spring water
3. Repurpose leftovers to make a new meal
4. Use steamers to reheat foods like grains
5. Reheat the food the same way it was cooked, for example if you prepared a bake or stir fry, reheat same way
6. Use oven-safe storage containers for easier reheating straight out of storage in the refrigerator
7. Use a toaster oven
8. Invest in a crock-pot
9. When reheating, wrap some foods in foil first
10. Finally, take off your microwave from your kitchen. What other way to avoid using something other than taking it out of sight and out of reach?

Dealing with Leftovers

If you can't feed them to your pets or use them in compost, either throw them away or use your creativity and a little bit of additional spice or ingredients to turn them into tasty snacks. Most leftovers can be reused after reheating and having something added to them which gives them "life."

10 ideas on how to use leftovers:

1. A vegetable or fruit can be used for breakfast by being added to your muesli or smoothie. Alternatively, you can have it as a snack later in the day.

2. Bananas that start to go brown should be peeled and put in freezer bags. After defrosting, mash them and add them to smoothies or cake batter.

3. Leftover flat bread can be ground into breadcrumbs and frozen. You can use it later for a coating for fried foods, or use it as a crunchy substitute for granola in parfaits.

4. Lettuce or Kale leaves going limp can be stir-fried.

5. If you have a little bit of leftover mustard, add some white wine vinegar, honey, and olive oil into the jar, season to taste, replace the lid, and shake well. You will get a great salad dressing.

6. Apples going soft can be cored and filled with dried fruits, or nuts. Bake them for 20 minutes and you'll get a healthy and tasty dessert.

7. Leftover herbs can be turned into a dressing. Chop and mix them with key lime juice and olive oil. Season to taste and chill before serving.

8. Leftover dried fruit and nuts. Add them to cooked and fluffed-up rice together with some fresh herbs and key lime juice.

9. Leftover pitta or tortilla wraps can be turned into delicious crisps. Break them into small pieces, lay them on a baking sheet, and drizzle with a little bit of avocado oil and sea salt. Grill until they turn golden brown at the edges. Serves as crisp or scatter over salad.

10. Leftover cooked rice can be reused if you fry 1 chopped onion in a little bit of avocado oil and add some onion powder. Mix well, add the cooked rice. Wait for a few minutes, add chopped veggies, and serve warm.

Chapter 2

The Progressive Dr. Sebi Meal Prep Guideline

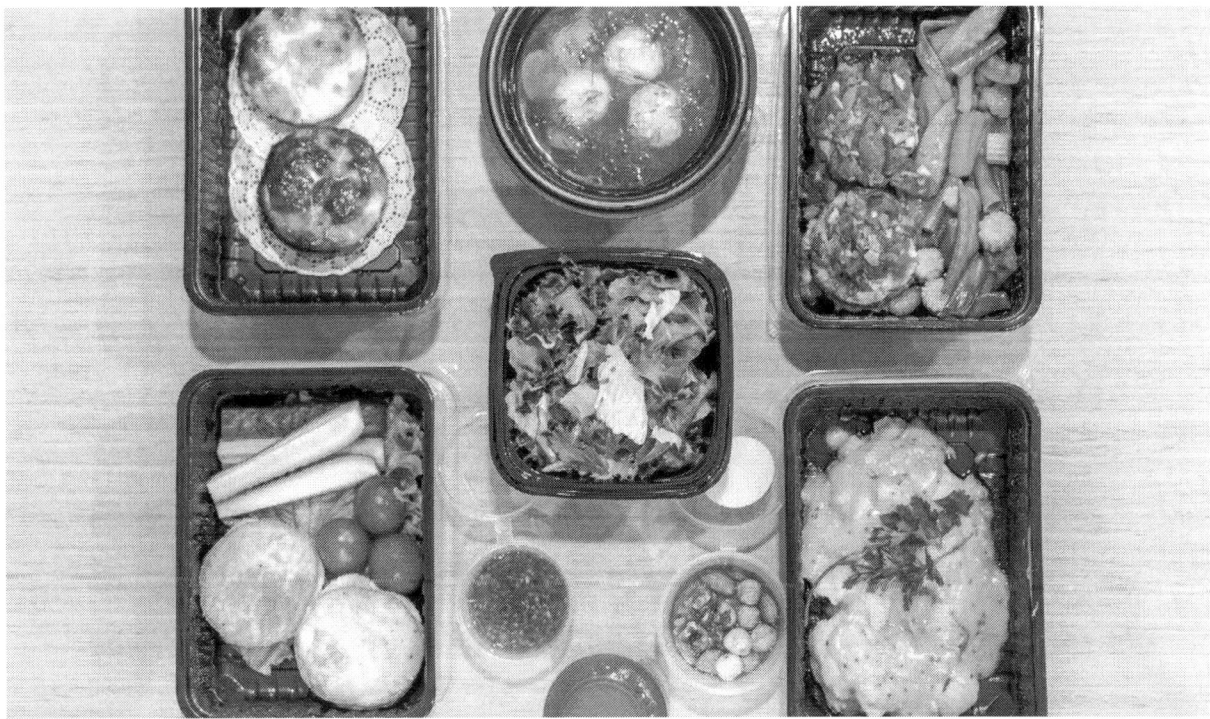

A meal prep guideline is there to help you organize your life in a way that will ensure you always eat healthy meals without having to spend a lot of time preparing them.

Meal Planning

Generally speaking, meal planning makes your life easier especially if you're on a diet that requires sticking to a specific eating plan. In the case of Dr. Sebi Alkaline diet, there is a list of foods that are allowed and those that are not. This actually makes your meal prepping very easy because there is a limited list of foods approved by Dr. Sebi so all you have to do is shop according to this list. Besides, as Dr. Sebi diet is practically a vegan diet, the focus is on fruits and vegetables so meal prepping revolves around soups, salads, smoothies, juices, and steamed vegetables. Although this may not always possible, it's best to use foods that are in season. However, some of the foods in the Dr. Sebi Food List are not available everywhere so you may have to substitute them with similar food provided they are included on the Dr. Sebi Food List (e.g. you can substitute avocado with nuts). The main purpose of meal planning is to make you think strategically about your diet and to shop according to a shopping list based on Dr. Sebi-approved foods. The basics of meal prepping is meal planning which starts with selecting the recipes, deciding how many meals you are going to prepare (e.g. three meals per day or just one, the main one), and for how many days you want to plan ahead. Although planning is only the first step, it is the most important one.

Shopping for Ingredients

Once you have an idea of what meals you are going to prepare and for how many days, you should make a shopping list. If you are meal prepping for several other people besides yourself, you may have to consider their preferences. This makes meal prepping slightly more difficult but at least you'll make sure everyone eats what they like.

When shopping for ingredients you also need to consider how many meals you are going to prepare. The more meals, the more it pays to buy in bulk.
You can do your shopping on a Friday afternoon on your way home from work, or anytime during the week or weekend if that suits your lifestyle. However, if you're not used to cooking large quantities of food, you may start by cooking for only two days ahead until you become better-organized.

Meal Prepping Basics

Meal prepping starts with meal planning and food shopping. The tricky part starts when you get home and have to organize all the ingredients, prepare them, cook them, and finally store them to be used at a later date. The very thought of having to spend several hours cooking for a week ahead may be enough to put people off the meal prepping idea. If you are new to this, the first thing you should do when you get home and unload all the food on your countertop is to have a cup of herbal tea (that surely will calm you down). Change into more comfortable clothes, put on some nice music, and you're ready to start. Then, if you haven't done so already, clean out your fridge and throw out all the foods that are beyond the "use by" date. Clean the fridge if you need to.

Put the perishables and foods you will not be cooking that day in the fridge as soon as you get home, e.g. lettuce, fruits, etc. Besides, you should try to avoid as many distractions while you're cooking as that will only prolong the time you spend in the kitchen (e.g. don't read your emails or SMSs, don't even answer the phone, etc.).

Once you're ready, start cleaning, rinsing, chopping, grating, boiling, and sorting. When meal prepping becomes a routine, it won't take a lot of time. There's something else to consider. Our thoughts affect our emotions and behavior and according to Ayurveda, it's particularly important not to be in a bad mood when cooking. To those who are not familiar with the philosophy of Ayurveda, this may come as a surprise, but most women will confirm that, if possible, you should refrain from cooking or baking if feeling resentful, angry, stressed or exhausted. They may not have heard of Ayurveda but they know that emotions and thoughts DO affect the final result.

Why do I mention this? If you have to cook for a big family or family members with different diets and preferences and you are the only one who has to do the shopping, cooking, and cleaning afterward, you may often feel unappreciated. The trouble is that the resentment and bitterness which you are unaware of may find its way to your meals. I know that might sound cheeky but it is what it is. When feeling this way, either ask someone else to do the cooking or postpone the cooking for another day when your mind is not flooded with negative thoughts.

Meal Prepping Workflow

Meal prepping starts with preparing ingredients for different meals. The more meals you plan to prepare, the better organized you need to be when it comes to shopping, cooking, and storing. What helps is preparing meals in a specific order.

A well-thought-through workflow can save you a lot of time. Choose which meals to cook first based on cook times. Before you start cooking, check if you have all the ingredients you had planned to use that day. You should have selected recipes beforehand, i.e. before you have done the shopping.

Once prepared, meals should be cooled and stored - in the fridge, if you plan to use them in the next couple of days or the freezer if you plan on using them at a much later date.

Tips for a well-organized workflow:

- **Slow Cooker first**

Start with meals that require the longest cook time. Although food cooked in slow cookers takes a long time to cook, cooking this way saves you time because if your cooker has an automatic timer, all you have to do is set it to a certain time. Foods cooked "low and slow" also tend to retain more nutrients. However, cooking in a slow cooker may take as long as 8 hours, so if cooking in bulk, it's best to start with a meal that should be cooked this way. While it cooks, you have plenty of time to cook all the other meals you had planned for that day.

- **Oven-cooked recipes next**

An oven needs some time to reach the desired temperature and although meals cooked in the oven generally taste better than those cooked on the stovetop, they usually take longer to cook. This is why they should be done immediately after the slow cooker meals. Or, if you are not using a slow cooker, start by preparing the meal that needs to be cooked in the oven first.

- **Stove Top recipes to follow**

Once the slow-cooker and oven-cooked meals are underway, you can focus on meals cooked on the stovetop, which is where most of the meals are prepared. Meals that are only partly cooked and that will be cooked at a later date may take as little 10 minutes cook time. Others that need to be cooked thoroughly, will take an hour or so.

- **No-Bake recipes to follow**

Cold meals are usually done last and you can start with them only once other meals are cooking or have already been cooked and are cooling.

- **Putting it all together**

To make it easier to stick to the Dr. Sebi Alkaline Diet plan, start meal prepping so that you always have Dr. Sebi approved meals ready even if you don't feel like cooking or come home too late to start cooking from scratch. Besides, don't forget that Dr. Sebi diet includes many herbs and herbal teas. When shopping for ingredients to use in your meals, make sure you don't run out of herbs and spices.

Chapter 3

Meal Prepping

Week 1 – Shopping List

Items:

- Agave syrup
- Apple sauce, homemade
- Arugula, 8 oz.
- Avocado
- Basil leaves
- Bromide Plus Powder
- Burro banana
- Cayenne pepper
- Cherry tomatoes, 1 pint
- Chickpeas, 15.5 oz.
- Cucumber, large
- Date sugar
- Dr. Sebi's Herbal Tea
- Dried thyme
- Grapeseed oil
- Green bell pepper
- Homemade applesauce
- Homemade vegetable broth
- Homemade walnut milk
- Kamut flour tortilla
- Key lime
- Mango, large
- Nori sheets
- Olive oil
- Papaya, 1 lb.
- Peach, large
- Pitted dates
- Quinoa, 8.5 oz.
- Raisins
- Red onion, large, count 1
- Sea salt
- Sesame seeds
- Sliced white mushrooms, 8 oz.
- Soft-jelly coconut
- Soft-jelly coconut water
- Spelt flour, 680 g
- Spring water
- Sprouted hemp seeds
- Tahini butter
- Walnut halves, 7.5 ounces
- Whole Berry Medley, 16 oz.
- Wild rice, 16 oz.
- Zucchini, large

Week 1

Day 1
Breakfast – Herbal Smoothie

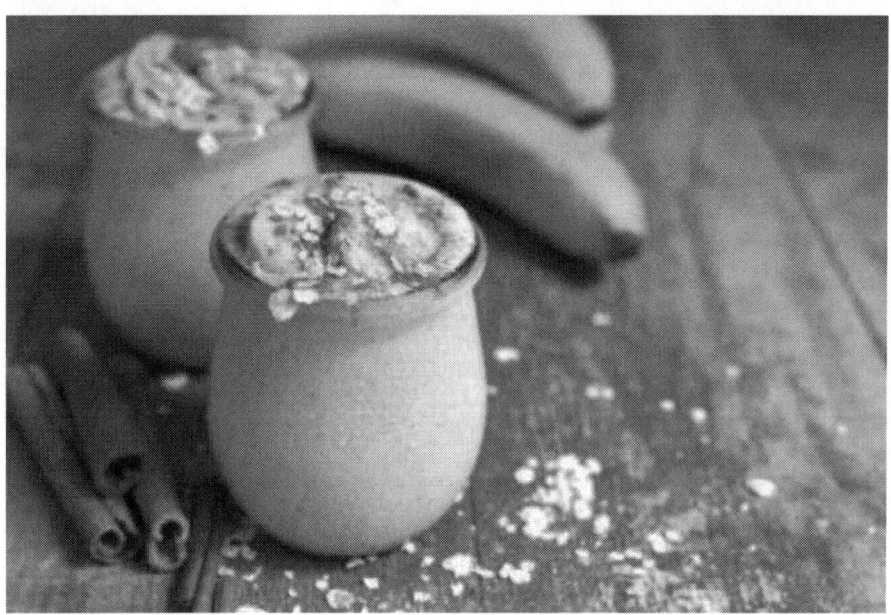

Serving: 2

Preparation time: 5 minutes; Cooking time: 0 minutes;
Nutritional Info: 75.5 Cal; 2.1 g Fats; 0.9 g Protein; 13.2 g Carb; 1.8 g Fiber;

Ingredients

- 2 cups Dr. Sebi's Herbal Tea
- 1 burro banana, peeled
- 1 tablespoon walnut
- 1 tablespoon agave syrup

Directions

1. Plug in a high-speed food processor or blender and add all the ingredients in its jar.
2. Cover the blender jar with its lid and then pulse for 40 to 60 seconds until smooth.
3. Divide the drink between two glasses and then serve.

Storage instructions:

Divide drink between two jars or bottles, cover with a lid and then store the containers in the refrigerator for up to 3 days.

Lunch – Mushroom Risotto

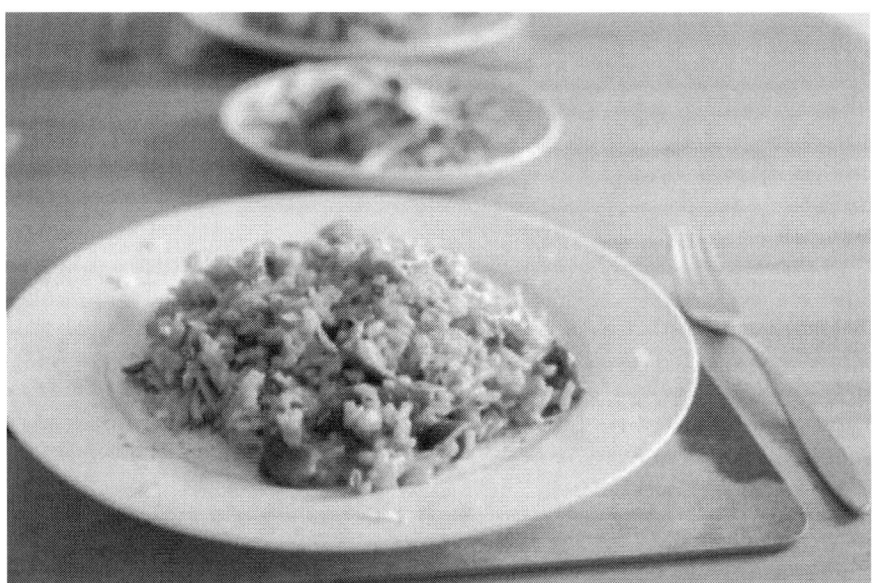

Serving: 2

Preparation time: 5 minutes; Cooking time: 1 hour and 25 minutes;
Nutritional Info: 133 Cal; 1.3 g Fats; 4.5 g Protein; 25.2 g Carb; 2.4 g Fiber;

Ingredients

- 4 ounces sliced mushrooms
- ¼ of an onion, chopped
- 1 cup wild rice
- 1 tablespoon grapeseed oil
- 2 cups vegetable broth, homemade
- 1/3 teaspoon salt
- ¼ teaspoon cayenne pepper

Directions

1. Take a medium pot, place it over medium heat add oil and when hot, add onion and mushroom and then cook for 4 to 5 minutes until mushrooms have turned golden brown and the liquid in the pan have evaporated.
2. Add rice, stir until mixed, cook for 1 minute, and then stir in salt and cayenne pepper.
3. Pour in the broth, switch heat to the low level and then cook the rice for 1 hour and 20 minutes until rice is tender and then serve.

Storage instructions:

Cool the meal, divide evenly between two meal prep containers, cover with a lid, and then store the containers in the refrigerator for up to 7 days.

Reheating instructions:

When ready to eat, reheat in the oven for 1 to 2 minutes until hot and then serve.

Dinner – Pesto Zoodles

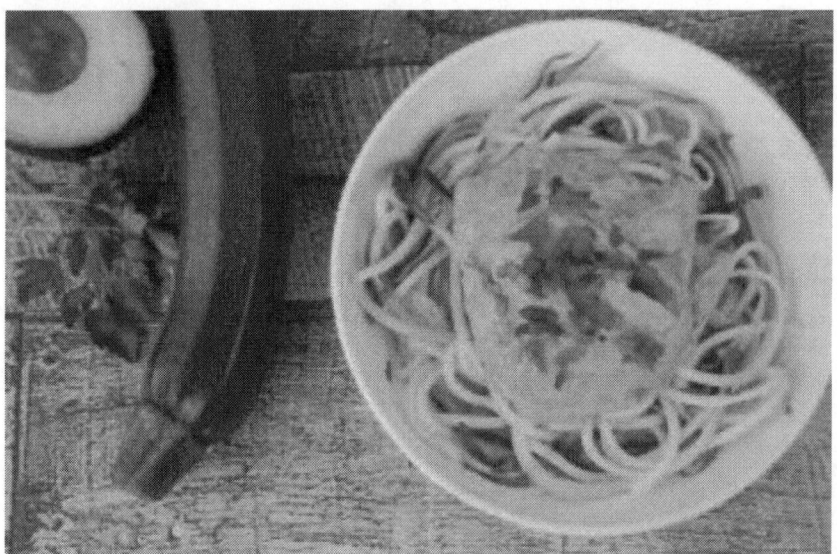

Serving: 2; Preparation time: 10 minutes; Cooking time: 5 minutes;

Nutritional Info: 214 Cal; 1017.10 g Fats; 4.8 g Protein; 13.2 g Carb; 6.1 g Fiber;

Ingredients

- 2 zucchini
- 1 avocado, peeled, pitted
- ½ cup cherry tomatoes
- 2 tablespoons walnuts
- ½ of key lime, juiced
- ¼ teaspoon salt; 1/8 teaspoon cayenne pepper
- 2 teaspoons grapeseed oil
- 2 tablespoons olive oil

Directions

1. Prepare the zucchini noodles and for this, cut them into thin strips by using a vegetable peeler or use a spiralizer.
2. Then take a medium skillet pan, add oil in it and when hot, add zucchini noodles in it and then cook for 3 to 5 minutes until tender-crisp.
3. Meanwhile, place the remaining ingredients in a food processor and then pulse until the creamy paste comes together.
4. When zucchini noodles have sautéed, drain and place them in a large bowl and add the blended sauce in it. Add 2 tablespoons of water and then toss until well combined. Garnish the zoodles with grated coconut.

Storage instructions:

Cool the meal, divide evenly between two meal prep containers, cover with a lid, and then store the containers in the refrigerator for up to 7 days.

Reheating instructions:

When ready to eat, reheat in the oven for 1 to 2 minutes until hot and then serve.

Day 2
Breakfast – Peach Muffin

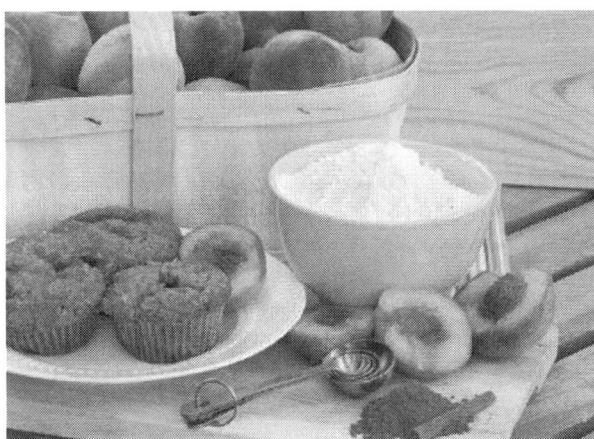

Serving: 2; **Preparation time: 10 minutes; Cooking time: 15 minutes;**

Nutritional Info: 76.1 Cal; 3.3 g Fats; 0.9 g Protein; 14.3 g Carb; 0.9 g Fiber;

Ingredients

- 2/3 cup spelt flour
- ½ of peach, chopped
- 1 teaspoon mashed burro banana
- 2/3 tablespoons chopped walnuts
- 6 ½ tablespoons walnut milk, homemade
- 1/16 teaspoon salt; 2 2/3 tablespoon date sugar
- 2/3 tablespoon spring water, warmed
- 2/3 teaspoon key lime juice

Directions

1. Switch on the oven, then set it to 400 degrees F and let it preheat.
2. Meanwhile, peel the peach, cut it in half, remove the pit and then cut one half of peach in ½-inch pieces, reserving the other half of peach for later use.
3. Take a medium bowl, pour in the milk, and then whisk in mashed banana and lime juice until well combined. Take a separate medium bowl, place flour in it, add salt and date sugar, stir until mixed, whisk in milk mixture until smooth, and then fold in peached until mixed. Take four silicone muffin cups, grease them with oil, fill them evenly with the prepared batter and then sprinkle walnuts on top.
4. Bake the muffins for 10 to 15 minutes until the top is nicely golden brown and inserted toothpick into each muffin comes out clean. When done, let muffins cool

Storage instructions:

Wrap each muffin in a plastic wrap and then store in the refrigerator for up to 7 days.

Reheating instructions:

When ready to eat, uncover the muffins, reheat in the oven for 1 to 2 minutes until hot and then serve.

Lunch – Energy Balls

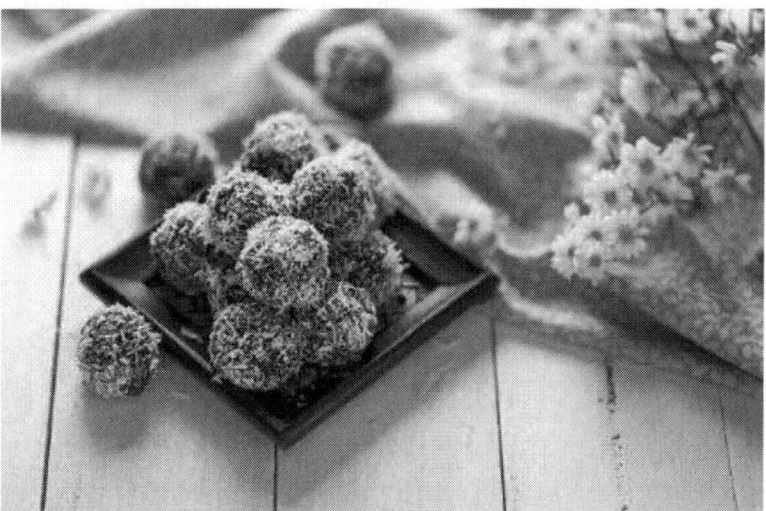

Serving: 2

Preparation time: 10 minutes; Cooking time: 0 minutes;
Nutritional Info: 119 Cal; 8 g Fats; 2 g Protein; 10 g Carb; 1 g Fiber;

Ingredients

- ¼ cup blueberries
- ¼ cup dried dates
- 1 cup soft-jelly coconut, shredded
- ¼ cup walnuts
- ½ teaspoon date sugar

Extra:

- ½ tablespoon agave syrup
- 1/16 teaspoon salt

Directions

1. Place walnuts in a food processor and then pulse until the mixture resembles a fine powder.
2. Then add berries, coconut, date sugar and dates, pulse until just mixed and then slowly blend in agave syrup until the soft paste comes together.
3. Spoon the mixture into a medium bowl, chill it for a minimum of 30 minutes and then roll the mixture into balls, 1 tablespoon of mixture per ball.
4. Roll the balls into some more coconut.

Storage instructions:

Place balls in an airtight container and store in the refrigerator for up to 5 days.

Reheating instructions:

When ready to eat, bring the balls to room temperature and then serve.

Dinner – Quinoa Bowl

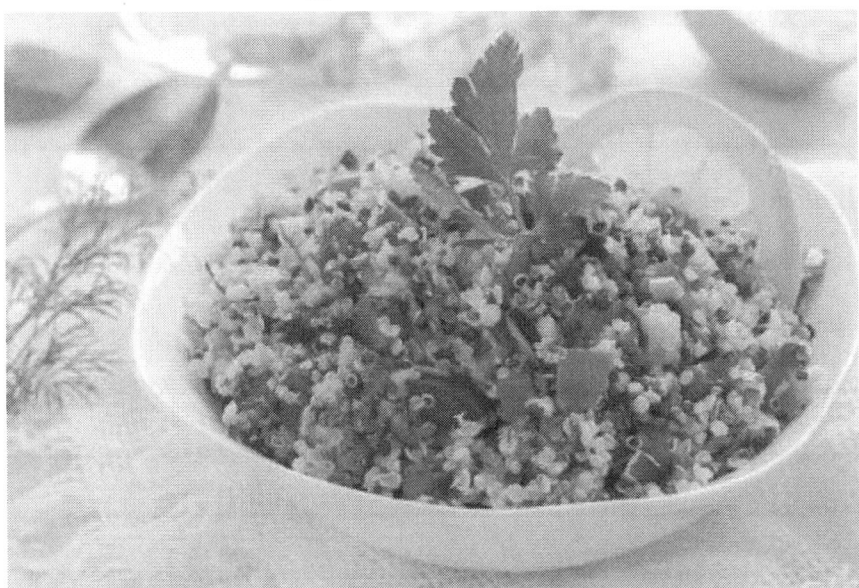

Serving: 2

Preparation time: 5 minutes; Cooking time: 3 minutes;
Nutritional Info: 141 Cal; 6.2 g Fats; 6.5 g Protein; 32 g Carb; 4.1 g Fiber;

Ingredients

- 1/3 cup quinoa, cooked
- ¼ cup cherry tomatoes, quartered
- ½ of green bell pepper, chopped
- 1/3 cup basil leaves
- 1 tablespoon grapeseed oil

Extra:

- ¼ teaspoon salt
- 1/8 teaspoon cayenne pepper

Directions

1. Take a skillet pan, place it over medium-high heat, add oil and when hot, add cherry tomatoes and bell pepper and cook for 2 to 3 minutes until tender-crisp.
2. Take a medium bowl, place cooked quinoa in it, add tomatoes and bell pepper mixture, and then add basil leaves.
3. Season with salt and cayenne pepper, stir until mixed.

Storage instructions:

Cool the meal, divide evenly between two meal prep containers, cover with a lid, and then store the containers in the refrigerator for up to 7 days.

Reheating instructions:

When ready to eat, reheat in the oven for 1 to 2 minutes until hot and then serve.

Day 3
Breakfast – Triple Berry Smoothie

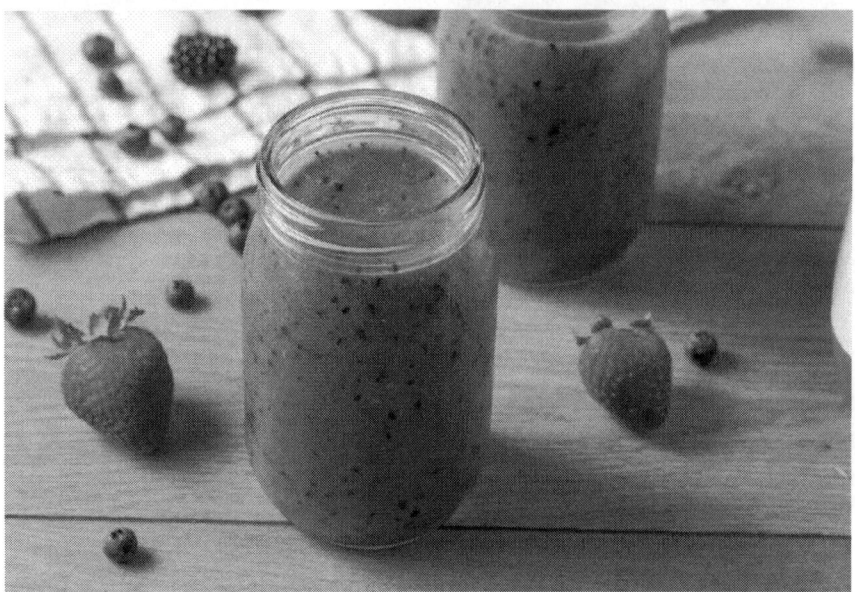

Serving: 2

Preparation time: 5 minutes; Cooking time: 0 minutes;
Nutritional Info: 130 Cal; 1.5 g Fats; 5 g Protein; 26 g Carb; 4 g Fiber;

Ingredients

- ½ cup strawberries
- 2 tablespoons agave syrup
- ½ cup raspberries
- 1 burro banana, peeled
- ½ cup blueberries
- 1 cup spring water

Directions

1. Plug in a high-speed food processor or blender and add all the ingredients in its jar.
2. Cover the blender jar with its lid and then pulse for 40 to 60 seconds until smooth.
3. Divide the drink between two glasses and then serve.

Storage instructions:

Divide drink between two jars or bottles, cover with a lid and then store the containers in the refrigerator for up to 3 days.

Lunch – Spelt and Raisin Cookies

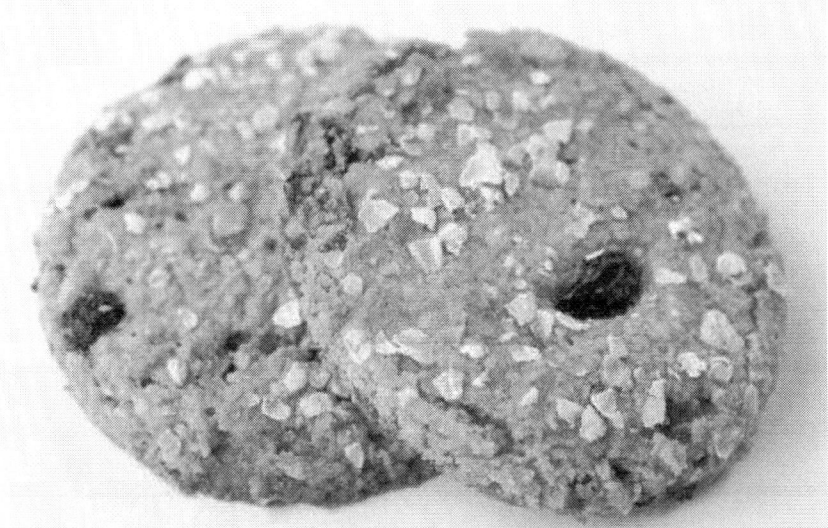

Serving: 2

Preparation time: 10 minutes; Cooking time: 18 minutes;
Nutritional Info: 149.2 Cal; 4 g Fats; 3 g Protein; 55.3 g Carb; 2.2 g Fiber;

Ingredients

- 1 cup spelt flour
- 1/3 cup raisins
- ½ cup dates, pitted
- 3 ½ tablespoons, applesauce homemade or pureed apples
- 2/3 tablespoon spring water

Extra:

- 1/16 teaspoon sea salt
- 2 tablespoons agave syrup
- 1 ¾ tablespoon grapeseed oil

Directions

1. Switch on the oven, then set it to 350 degrees F and let it preheat.
2. Meanwhile, place flour in a food processor, add dates and salt in it, and then pulse until well blended.
3. Transfer flour mixture into a medium bowl, add remaining ingredients, and then stir until well mixed.
4. Divide the mixture into parts, each part about 2 tablespoons of the mixture, and then shape each part into a ball.
5. Place the cookie ball on a cookie sheet lined with parchment sheet, flatten it slightly by using a fork and then bake for 18 minutes until done.
6. Let cookies cool for 10 minutes and then serve.

Storage instructions:

Place cookies in an airtight container and store for up to 7 days.

Dinner – Salad Burritos

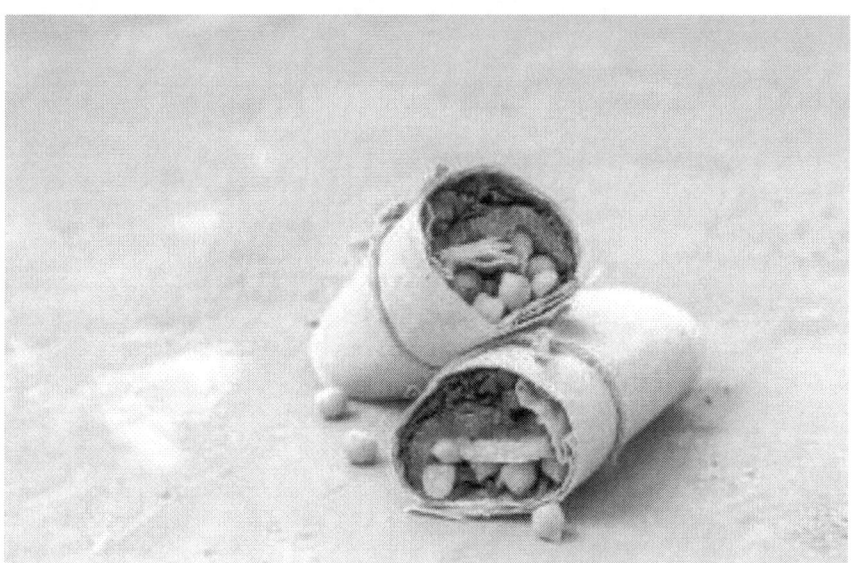

Serving: 2

Preparation time: 10 minutes; Cooking time: 5 minutes;
Nutritional Info: 274 Cal; 9.1 g Fats; 11.5 g Protein; 39 g Carb; 4.4 g Fiber;

Ingredients

- 2 ounces arugula
- ¼ cup cherry tomatoes
- 2 tablespoons tahini butter, homemade
- ¾ cup cooked chickpeas
- 2 Kamut flour tortillas

Extra:

- 1 tablespoon key lime juice
- ¼ teaspoon salt
- ¼ teaspoon cayenne pepper

Directions

1. Prepare the dressing and for this, take a small bowl, place tahini butter in it and then stir in lime juice until mixed.
2. Take a medium bowl, place tomatoes in it, add arugula and chickpeas, drizzle with the dressing, toss until mixed, then cover the bowl and let it rest in the refrigerator for 20 minutes.
3. When ready to eat, heat the tortillas until warm, fill them with chickpeas mixture, sprinkle with salt and cayenne pepper, and then roll to serve.

Storage instructions:

Wrap each wrap in plastic wrap and foil and then store in refrigerator for up to 3 days.

Reheating instructions:

When ready to eat, bring wrap to the room temperature or reheat in the oven for 1 to 2 minutes until hot and then serve.

Day 4
Breakfast – Blueberry Smoothie

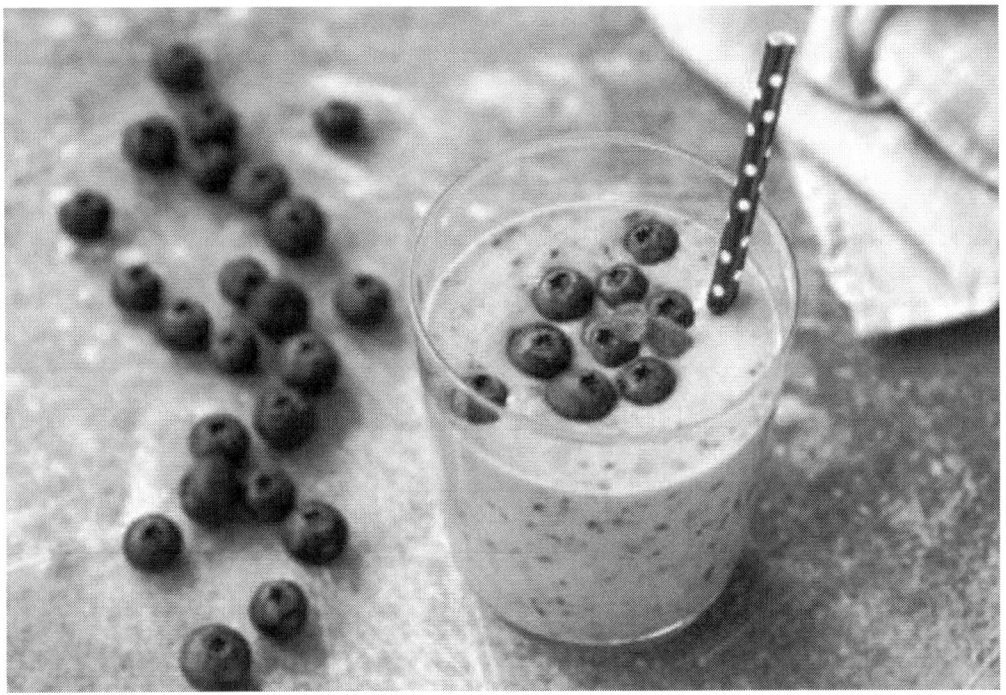

Serving: 2

Preparation time: 5 minutes; Cooking time: 0 minutes;
Nutritional Info: 194 Cal; 5 g Fats; 5 g Protein; 34 g Carb; 2 g Fiber;

Ingredients

- ½ cup blueberries
- 1 burro banana, peeled
- ¼ cup cooked quinoa
- 2 tablespoon date sugar
- 1 cup walnut milk, homemade

Directions

1. Plug in a high-speed food processor or blender and add all the ingredients in its jar.
2. Cover the blender jar with its lid and then pulse for 40 to 60 seconds until smooth.
3. Divide the drink between two glasses and then serve.

Storage instructions:

Divide drink between two jars or bottles, cover with a lid and then store the containers in the refrigerator for up to 3 days.

Lunch – Mango Salad

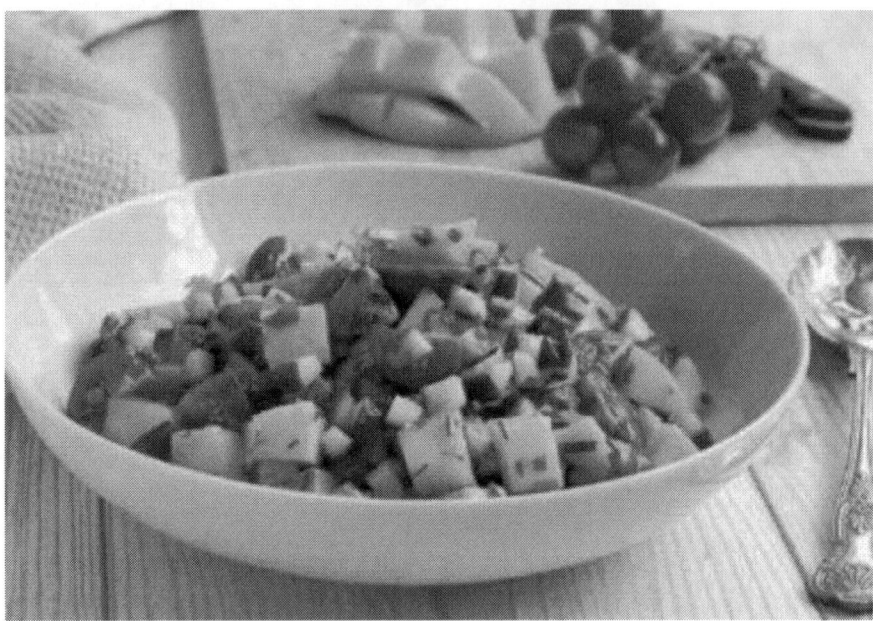

Serving: 2

Preparation time: 10 minutes; Cooking time: 0 minutes;
Nutritional Info: 108 Cal; 0.5 g Fats; 1 g Protein; 28.1 g Carb; 3.3 g Fiber;

Ingredients

- 1 mango, peeled, destoned, cubed
- ¼ of onion, chopped
- ½ cup cherry tomatoes, halved
- ½ of cucumber, deseeded, sliced
- ½ of green bell pepper, deseeded, sliced

Extra:

- 1/3 teaspoon salt
- ¼ teaspoon cayenne pepper
- ¼ of key lime, juiced

Directions

1. Take a medium bowl, place the mango pieces in it, add onion, tomatoes, cucumber, and bell pepper and then drizzle with lime juice.
2. Season with salt and cayenne pepper, toss until combined, and let the salad rest in the refrigerator for a minimum of 20 minutes.

Storage instructions:

Divide salad between two meal prep containers, cover with a lid, and then store the containers in the refrigerator for up to 3 days.

Dinner – Chickpea and Quinoa Burgers

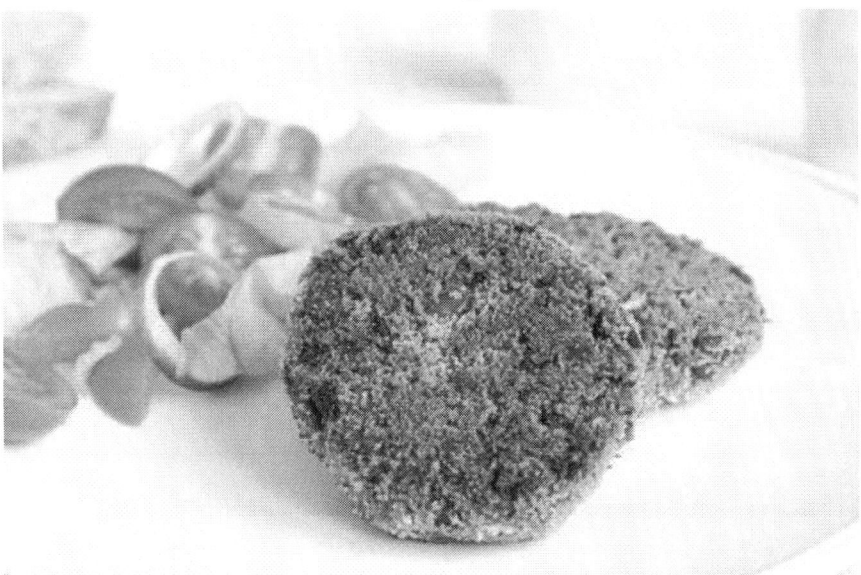

Serving: 2; Preparation time: 10 minutes; Cooking time: 20 minutes;

Nutritional Info: 315.4 Cal; 9.4 g Fats; 10.1 g Protein; 47.7 g Carb; 5.8 g Fiber;

Ingredients

- 2 tablespoons chopped onion
- ¾ cup chickpeas
- ¼ cup cooked quinoa
- 1 tablespoon spring water
- 1 tablespoon grapeseed oil
- 1/3 teaspoon salt
- 1/4 teaspoon cayenne pepper

Directions

1. Switch on the oven, then set it to 375 degrees F and let it preheat.
2. Meanwhile, place onion, chickpeas, quinoa into a food processor and then pulse little chunky mixture comes together.
3. Add water, salt, and cayenne pepper and then pulse until the dough comes together.
4. Then tip the mixture into a medium bowl, cover it with its lid and then let it rest in the refrigerator for 15 minutes.
5. Shape the mixture into two patties, place them on a baking sheet lined with parchment paper and then bake for 20 minutes, turning halfway.
6. Then switch on the broiler and continue cooking for 2 minutes per side until golden brown. You can serve the patties with spelt flour burgers and tahini butter.

Storage instructions:

Cool the patties, divide evenly between two oven-safe meal prep containers, cover with a lid, and then store the containers in the refrigerator for up to 7 days.

Reheating instructions:

When ready to eat, reheat in the oven for 1 to 2 minutes until hot and then serve as a burger.

Day 5
Breakfast – Raspberry, Peach and Walnuts Smoothie

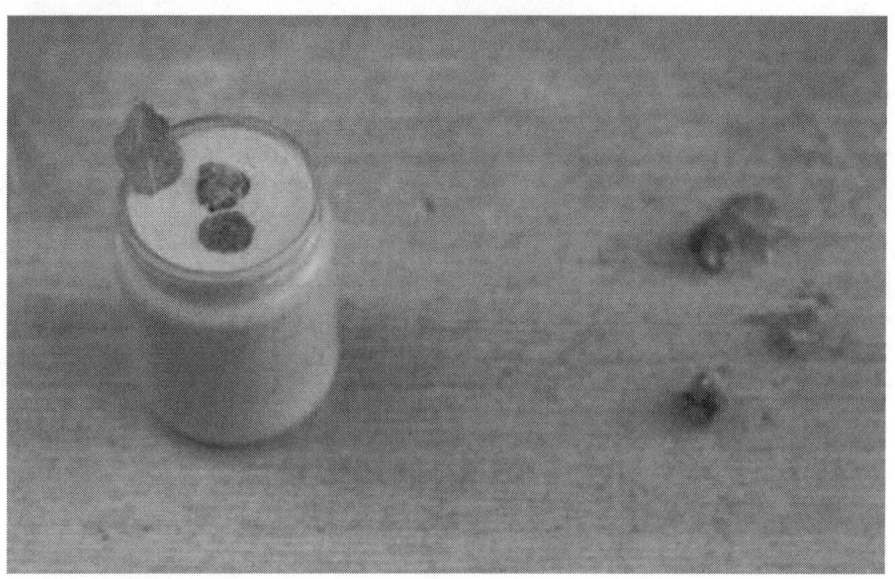

Serving: 2

Preparation time: 5 minutes; Cooking time: 0 minutes;
Nutritional Info: 165 Cal; 0.3 g Fats; 12 g Protein; 18.7 g Carb; 2.5 g Fiber;

Ingredients

- ½ of peach
- ½ cup raspberries
- 1 ½ tablespoons walnuts
- 2 tablespoons agave syrup
- ½ tablespoon Bromide Plus Powder
- 2 cups spring water

Extra:

- ¼ teaspoon salt
- 1/8 teaspoon cayenne pepper

Directions

1. Plug in a high-speed food processor or blender and add all the ingredients in its jar.
2. Cover the blender jar with its lid and then pulse for 40 to 60 seconds until smooth.
3. Divide the drink between two glasses and then serve.

Storage Instructions:

Divide drink between two jars or bottles, cover with a lid and then store the containers in the refrigerator for up to 3 days.

Lunch – Smoothie with Strawberries and Coconut

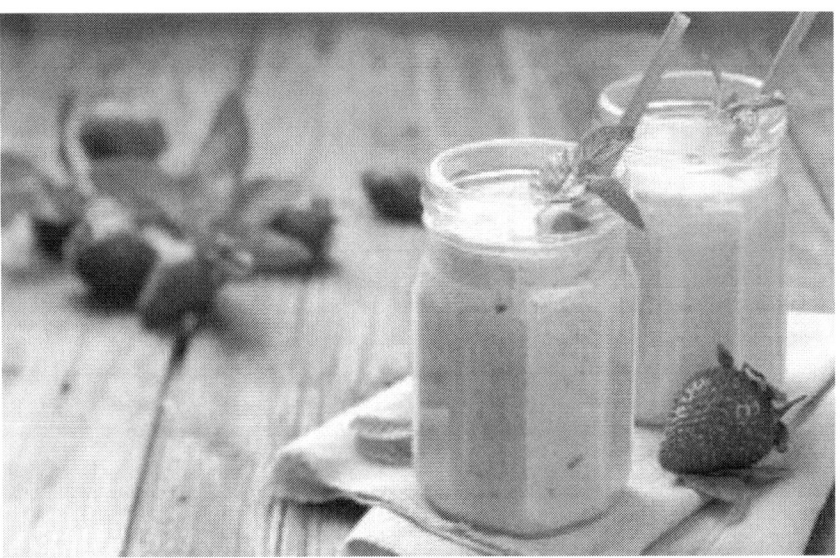

Serving: 2

Preparation time: 5 minutes; Cooking time: 10 minutes;
Nutritional Info: 168 Cal; 2.5 g Fats; 2 g Protein; 38 g Carb; 4.5 g Fiber;

Ingredients

- 1 ½ cup Dr. Sebi's Herbal Tea
- ¼ cup soft-jelly coconut, shredded
- ½ cup strawberries
- 2 tablespoons agave syrup

Directions

1. Plug in a high-speed food processor or blender and add all the ingredients in its jar.
2. Cover the blender jar with its lid and then pulse for 40 to 60 seconds until smooth.
3. Divide the drink between two glasses and then serve.

Storage instructions:

Divide drink between two jars, cover and then store the containers in the refrigerator for up to 3 days.

Dinner – Mushroom Gravy

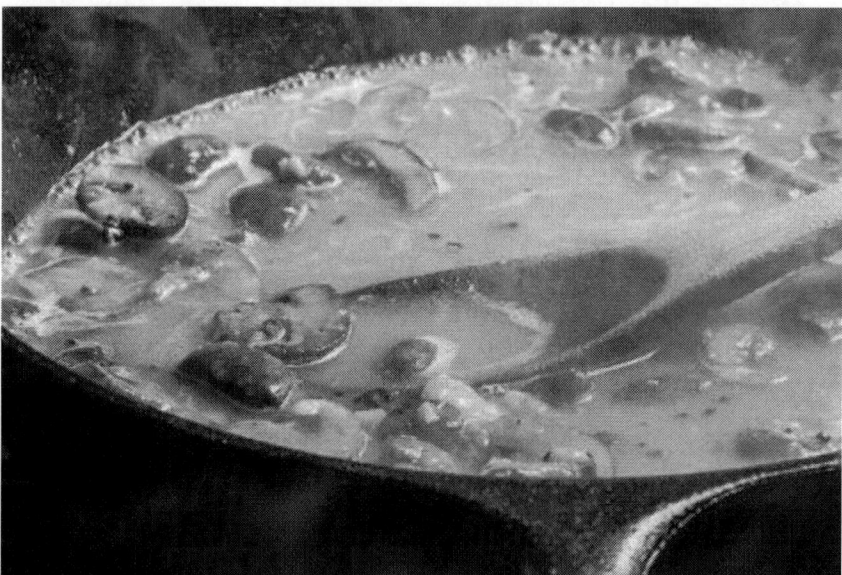

Serving: 2; Preparation time: 5 minutes; Cooking time: 12 minutes;

Nutritional Info: 65.3 Cal; 1.6 g Fats; 3.5 g Protein; 9.6 g Carb; 1 g Fiber;

Ingredients

- ¾ tablespoon spelt flour
- ¼ of onion, peeled, diced
- 4 ounces sliced mushrooms
- ½ cup walnut milk, homemade
- 1 tablespoon chopped walnuts
- ¼ teaspoon salt; 1/8 teaspoon cayenne pepper
- ½ teaspoon dried thyme
- 1 tablespoon grapeseed oil
- ¼ cup vegetable broth, homemade

Directions

1. Take a medium skillet pan, place it over medium heat, add oil and when hot, add onion and mushrooms, season with 1/16 teaspoon each of salt and cayenne pepper, and then cook for 4 minutes until tender.
2. Stir in spelt flour until coated, cook for 1 minute, slowly whisk in milk and vegetable broth and then season with remaining salt and cayenne pepper.
3. Switch heat to low-level, cook for 5 to 7 minutes until sauce has thickened slightly and then stir in walnuts and thyme.
4. Serve straight away with spelt flour bread.

Storage instructions:

Cool the meal, divide evenly between two meal prep containers, cover with a lid, and then store the containers in the refrigerator for up to 7 days.

Reheating instructions:

When ready to eat, reheat in the oven for 1 to 2 minutes until hot and then serve.

Day 6
Breakfast – Mineral Smoothie

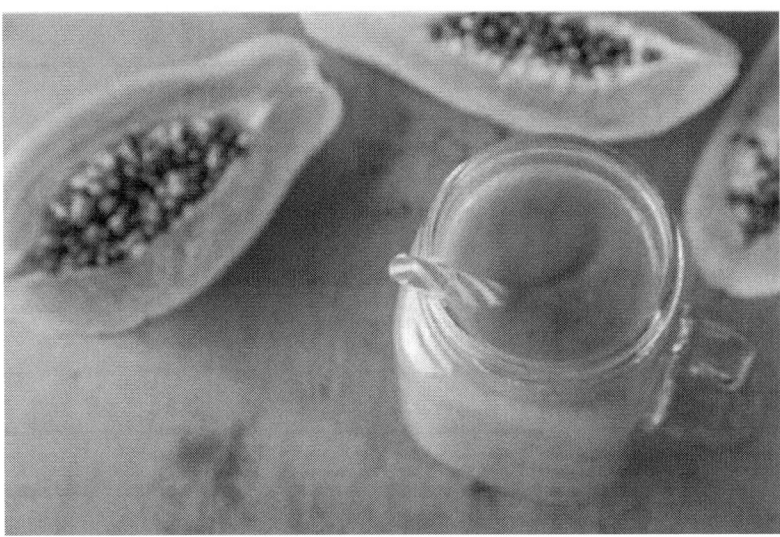

Serving: 2

Preparation time: 5 minutes; Cooking time: 0 minutes;
Nutritional Info: 152 Cal; 3.6 g Fats; 2.4 g Protein; 33 g Carb; 5 g Fiber;

Ingredients

- 1 papaya, deseeded
- 3 dates, pitted
- 1 burro banana, peeled
- ¼ of key lime, juiced
- 1 tablespoon Bromide Plus Powder

Extra:
- 1 cup spring water

Directions

1. Plug in a high-speed food processor or blender and add all the ingredients in its jar.
2. Cover the blender jar with its lid and then pulse for 40 to 60 seconds until smooth.
3. Divide the drink between two glasses and then serve.

Storage instructions:

Divide drink between two jars or bottles, cover with a lid and then store the containers in the refrigerator for up to 3 days.

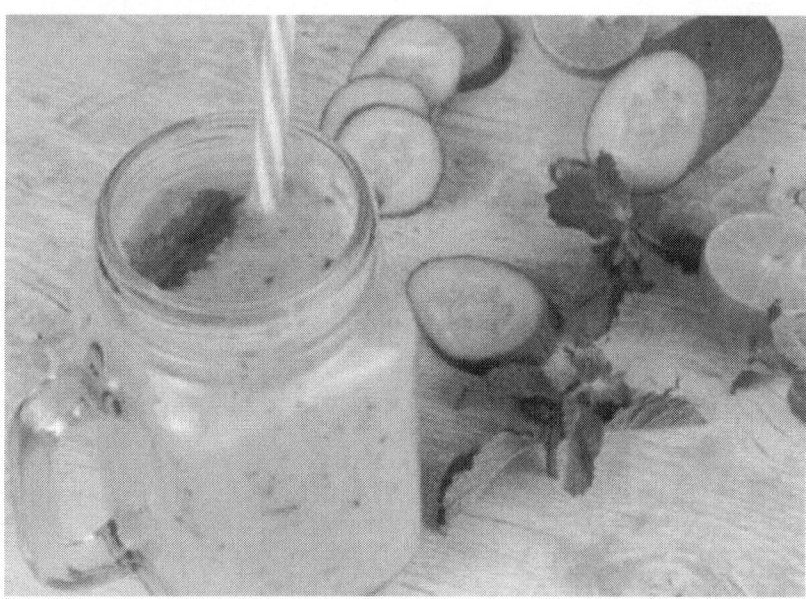

Lunch – Cucumber and Coconut Smoothie

Serving: 2

Preparation time: 5 minutes; Cooking time: 0 minutes;
Nutritional Info: 138 Cal; 5 g Fats; 3 g Protein; 22 g Carb; 3 g Fiber;

Ingredients

- 1 burro banana, peeled
- ½ of cucumber, deseeded
- ½ teaspoon Bromide Plus Powder
- ½ cup soft-jelly coconut water
- ½ cup Dr. Sebi's Herbal Tea

Directions

1. Plug in a high-speed food processor or blender and add all the ingredients in its jar.
2. Cover the blender jar with its lid and then pulse for 40 to 60 seconds until smooth.
3. Divide the drink between two glasses and then serve.

Storage instructions:

Divide drink between two jars or bottles, cover with a lid and then store the containers in the refrigerator for up to 3 days.

Dinner – Spring Salad

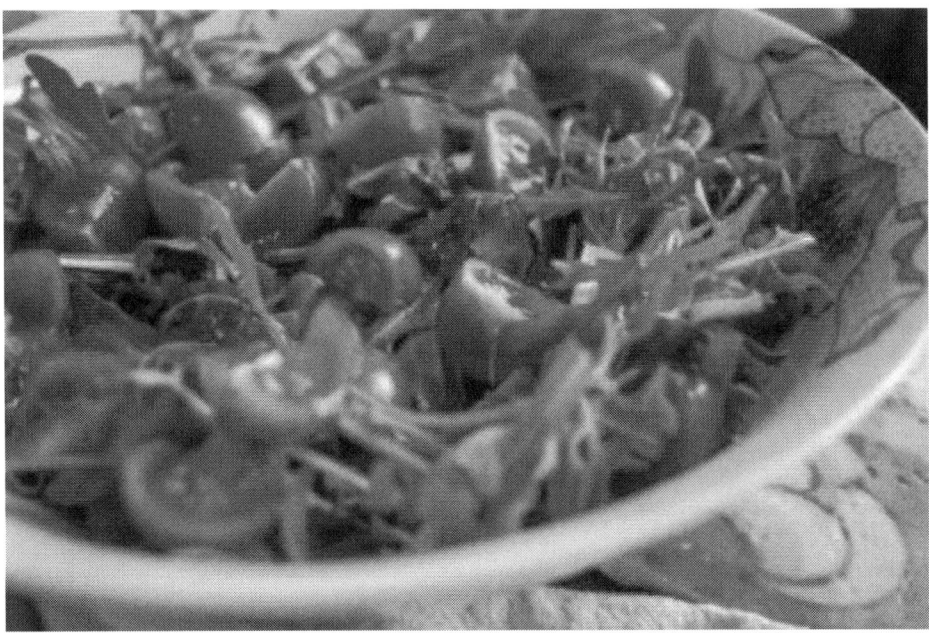

Serving: 2

Preparation time: 5 minutes; Cooking time: 10 minutes;
Nutritional Info: 87.3 Cal; 7 g Fats; 1.4 g Protein; 6 g Carb; 1.3 g Fiber;

Ingredients

- 4 ounces arugula
- ½ cup cherry tomatoes, halved
- ¼ cup basil leaves
- ½ key lime, juiced
- 2 tablespoons walnuts

Extra:

- ¼ teaspoon salt
- 1/8 teaspoon cayenne pepper
- ½ tablespoon tahini butter

Directions

1. Prepare the dressing and for this, take a small bowl, place key lime juice in it, add tahini butter, salt, and cayenne pepper and then whisk until combined.
2. Take a medium bowl, place arugula, tomatoes and basil leaves in it, pour in the dressing, and then massage by using your hands.
3. Let the salad rest for 20 minutes, then taste to adjust seasoning and then serve.

Storage instructions:

Divide the salad evenly between two meal prep containers, cover with a lid, and then store the containers in the refrigerator for up to 5 days.

Day 7
Breakfast – Tamarind Cucumber Breakfast Drink

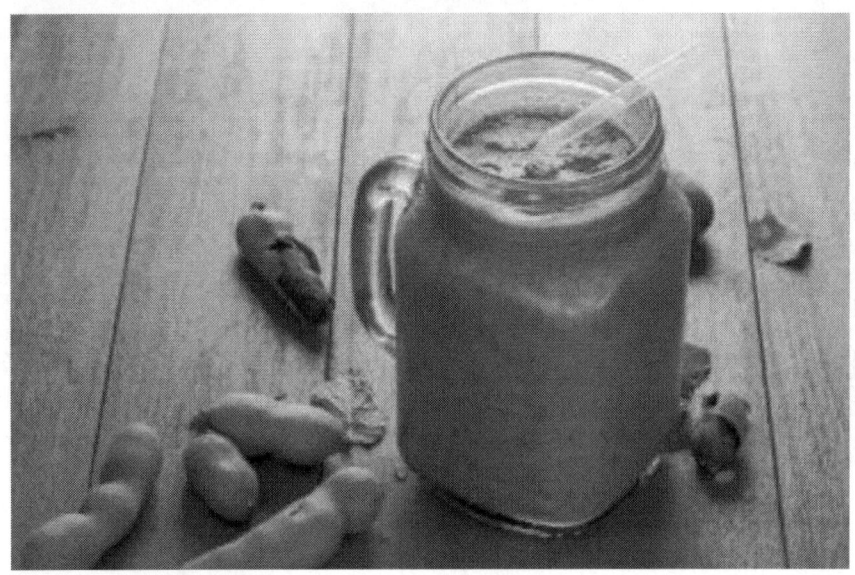

Serving: 2

Preparation time: 5 minutes; Cooking time: 0 minutes;
Nutritional Info: 110 Cal; 0.5 g Fats; 2 g Protein; 30.5 g Carb; 6.5 g Fiber;

Ingredients

- 2 cups Dr. Sebi's Herbal Tea
- 1 tablespoon tamarind pulp
- 1 cucumber, deseeded
- 2 ounces arugula
- 1 key lime, juiced

Extra:

- ¼ teaspoon salt
- 1/8 teaspoon cayenne pepper

Directions

1. Plug in a high-speed food processor or blender and add all the ingredients in its jar.
2. Cover the blender jar with its lid and then pulse for 40 to 60 seconds until smooth.
3. Divide the drink between two glasses and then serve.

Storage instructions:

Divide drink between two jars or bottles, cover with a lid and then store the containers in the refrigerator for up to 3 days.

Lunch – Raspberries Energy Balls

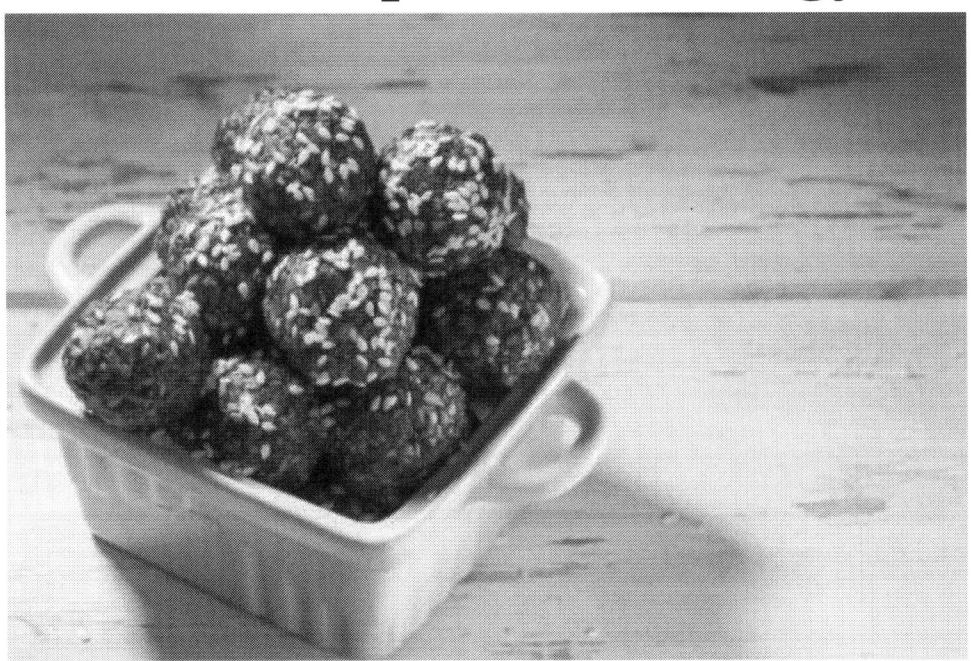

Serving: 2

Preparation time: 5 minutes; Cooking time: 0 minutes;
Nutritional Info: 123 Cal; 8 g Fats; 1 g Protein; 11 g Carb; 2 g Fiber;

Ingredients

- ½ cup raspberries
- 5 dates
- 1/16 teaspoon sea salt
- 1/3 cup walnuts
- 1 ½ cup soft-jelly coconut, shredded

Directions

1. Plug in a high-speed food processor or blender and add all the ingredients in its jar.
2. Cover the blender jar with its lid and then pulse for 40 to 60 seconds until well combined.
3. Shape the mixture into balls by using wet hands, 1 tablespoon of mixture per ball, place the balls on the tray, and let them freeze for a minimum of 30 minutes.
4. Serve straight away.

Storage instructions:

Store the balls in an airtight container and then store in the refrigerator for up to 7 days.

Reheating instructions:

When ready to eat, bring the balls to room temperature and then serve.

Dinner – Nori Burritos

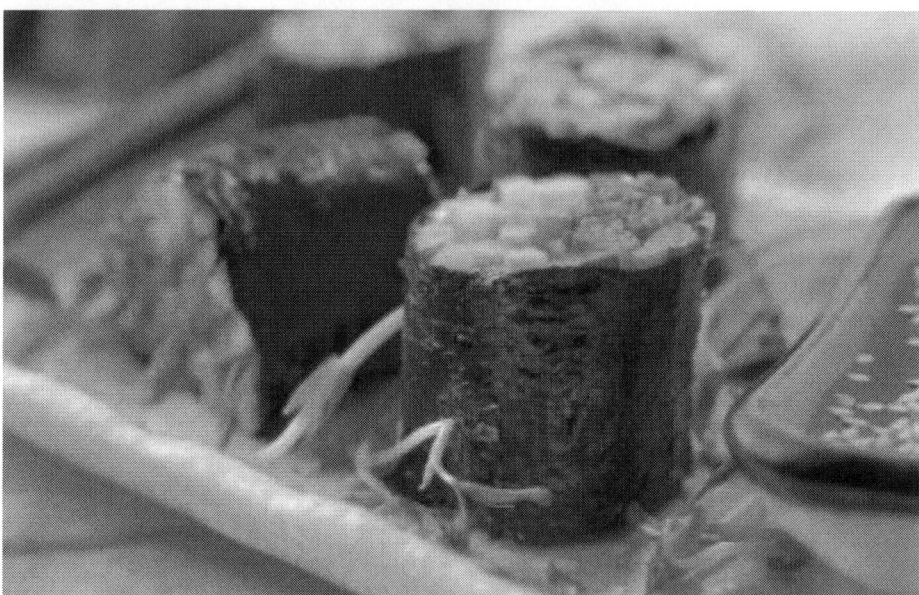

Serving: 2

Preparation time: 10 minutes; Cooking time: 0 minutes;
Nutritional Info: 90 Cal; 1.5 g Fats; 1.5 g Protein; 12.5 g Carb; 1 g Fiber;

Ingredients

- 1 avocado, peeled, sliced
- 1 cucumber, deseeded, cut into round slices
- 1 zucchini, sliced
- 2 teaspoons sprouted hemp seeds
- 2 nori sheets

Extra:

- 1 tablespoon tahini butter
- 2 teaspoons sesame seeds

Directions

1. Working on one nori sheet at a time, place it on a cutting board shiny-side-down and then arrange half of each avocado, cucumber and zucchini slices and tahini on it, leaving 1-inch wide spice to the right.
2. Then start folding the sheet over the fillings from the edge that is closest to you, cut into thick slices, and then sprinkle with 1 teaspoon of sesame seeds.
3. Repeat with the remaining nori sheet, and then serve.

Storage instructions:

Wrap each slice in a plastic wrap and foil and then refrigerate for up to 5 days.

Reheating instructions:

When ready to eat, unwrap the slices, bring to room temperature and then serve.

Week 2

Shopping List

Items:

- Agave syrup
- Amaranth greens
- Apple
- Arugula, 8 oz.
- Avocado
- Basil leaves
- Bromide Plus Powder
- Cayenne pepper
- Cherry tomatoes, 1 pint
- Chickpea flour
- Cucumber, large 1
- Dandelion greens
- Date sugar
- Dr. Sebi Herbal Tea
- Dried basil
- Figs
- Ginger Powder
- Grapeseed oil
- Homemade hummus
- Homemade walnut milk
- Iceberg lettuce
- Key lime
- Olive oil
- Onion powder
- Orange
- Oregano
- Purslane
- Red bell pepper
- Red onion, large
- Salt
- Sesame oil
- Sesame seeds
- Sliced white mushroom, 8 oz.
- Soft-jelly coconut milk
- Soft-jelly coconut water
- Spelt flour tortillas
- Spelt noodles
- Spring water
- Wakame stems
- Walnut butter
- Walnut halves, 7.5 ounces
- Whole Berry Medley, 16 oz.
- Zucchini

Day 1
Breakfast – Hearty Berry Smoothie

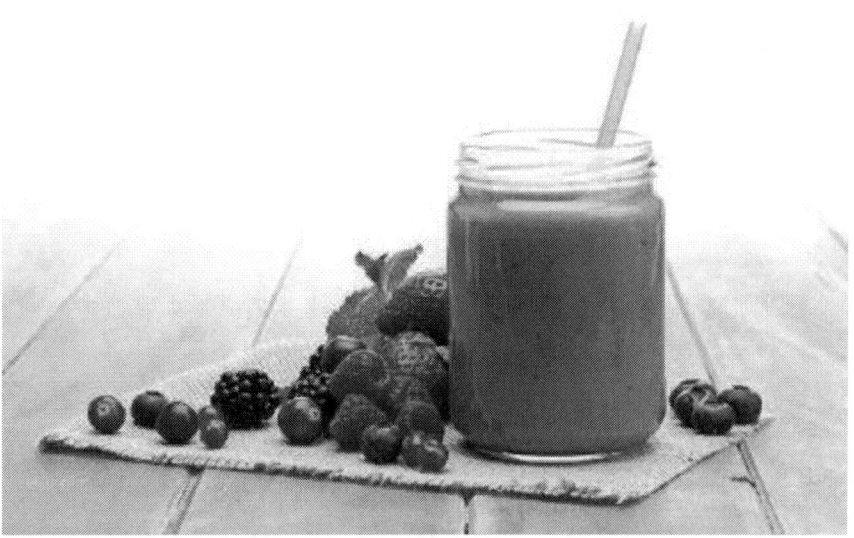

Serving: 2

Preparation time: 5 minutes; Cooking time: 0 minutes;
Nutritional Info: 180 Cal; 8 g Fats; 4 g Protein; 25 g Carb; 5 g Fiber;

Ingredients

- ¼ cup strawberries
- ¼ cup blueberries
- ¼ cup blackberries
- ¼ cup raspberries
- 2 tablespoons walnuts

Extra:

- 1 tablespoon of Bromide Plus Powder
- 2/3 cup spring water

Directions

1. Plug in a high-speed food processor or blender and add all the ingredients in its jar.
2. Cover the blender jar with its lid and then pulse for 40 to 60 seconds until smooth.
3. Divide the drink between two glasses and then serve.

Storage instructions:

Divide drink between two jars or bottles, cover with a lid and then store the containers in the refrigerator for up to 3 days.

Lunch – Cucumber and Arugula Salad

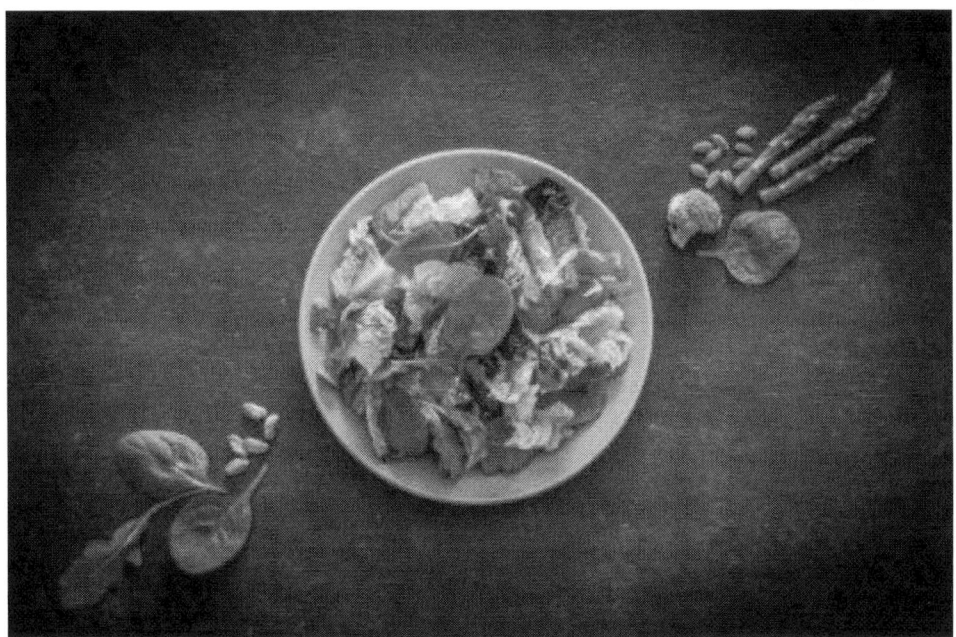

Serving: 2

Preparation time: 5 minutes; Cooking time: 0 minutes;
Nutritional Info: 142 Cal; 12.5 g Fats; 1.6 g Protein; 7.8 g Carb; 1 g Fiber;

Ingredients

- ½ of cucumber, deseeded
- 4 ounces arugula
- 1/8 teaspoon salt
- 1 tablespoon key lime juice
- 1 tablespoon olive oil

Extra:

- 1/8 teaspoon cayenne pepper

Directions

1. Cut the cucumber into slices, add to a salad bowl and then add arugula in it.
2. Mix together lime juice and oil until combined, pour over the salad, and then season with salt and cayenne pepper.
3. Toss until mixed and then serve.

Storage instructions:

Divide the salad evenly between two containers, cover with a lid, and then store the containers in the refrigerator for up to 5 days.

Dinner – Tef Grain Burger

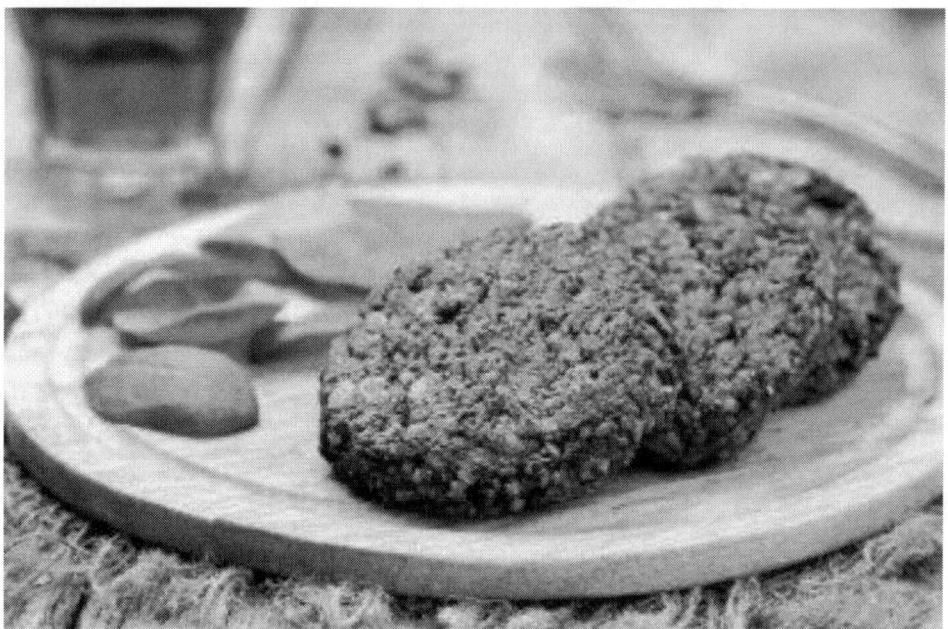

Serving: 2; Preparation time: 10 minutes; Cooking time: 8 minutes;

Nutritional Info: 122 Cal; 4.1 g Fats; 4.2 g Protein; 16.6 g Carb; 2.6 g Fiber;

Ingredients

- ¾ cup cooked tef grains
- ¾ cup chickpea flour
- 2 tablespoons diced onion
- 2 tablespoons diced red bell pepper
- ½ teaspoon dill
- ¼ teaspoon salt
- ½ teaspoon oregano
- 1/8 teaspoon cayenne pepper
- ½ teaspoon basil
- 1 tablespoon grapeseed oil

Directions

1. Take a medium pan, place over medium-heat, then add oil and when hot, add onion and bell pepper and cook for 3 minutes until tender.
2. Transfer vegetables into the large bowl, add remaining ingredients, stir until mixed, and then shape the mixture into patties.
3. Place patties into the pan and then cook for 3 minutes per side until crisp and golden brown on all sides. Serve straight away.

Storage instructions:

Cool the patties, divide evenly between two containers, cover with a lid, and then store the containers in the refrigerator for up to 7 days.

Reheating instructions:

When ready to eat, reheat in the oven for 1 to 2 minutes until hot and then serve.

Day 2
Breakfast – Green Smoothie

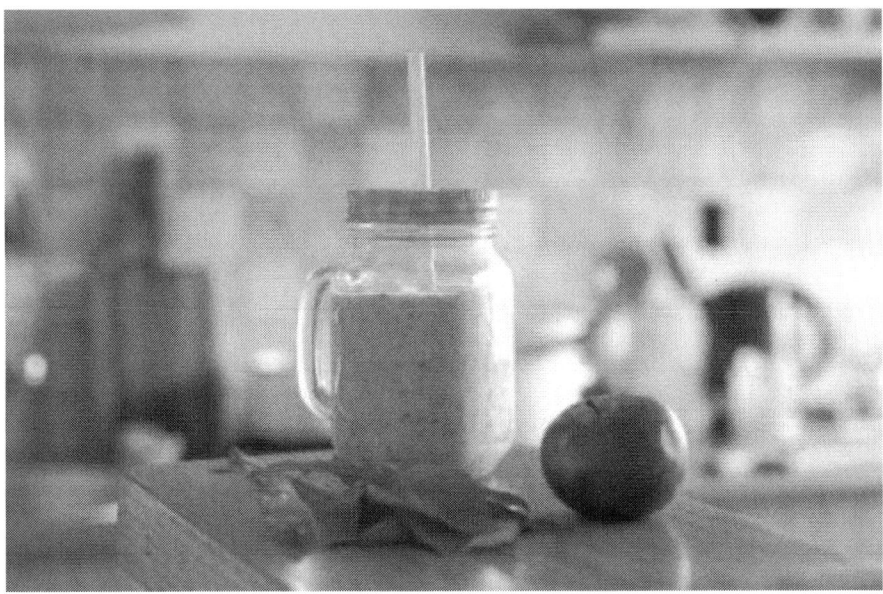

Serving: 2

Preparation time: 5 minutes; Cooking time: 0 minutes;
Nutritional Info: 317 Cal; 11 g Fats; 10 g Protein; 42 g Carb; 7 g Fiber;

Ingredients

- 1 cup dandelion greens
- ½ of cucumber, deseeded
- 1 apple, cored, deseeded
- 1 burro banana, peeled
- ½ tablespoon walnuts

Extra:

- ½ teaspoon Bromide Plus Powder
- 1 cup soft-jelly coconut milk

Directions

1. Plug in a high-speed food processor or blender and add all the ingredients in its jar.
2. Cover the blender jar with its lid and then pulse for 40 to 60 seconds until smooth.
3. Divide the drink between two glasses and then serve.

Storage instructions:

Divide drink between two bottles or jars, cover with their lids and then store the containers in the refrigerator for up to 3 days.

Lunch – Citrus Salad

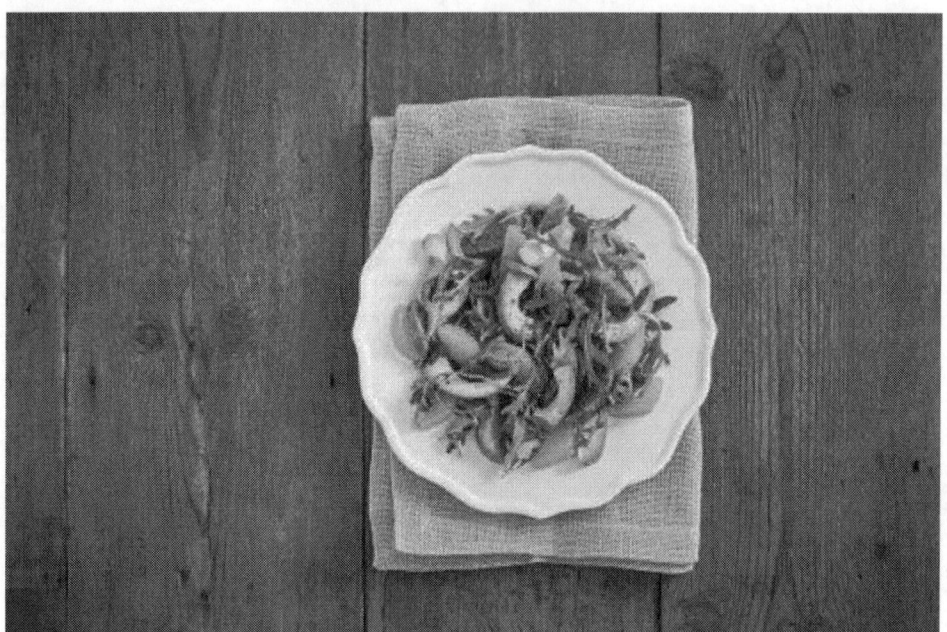

Serving: 2

Preparation time: 5 minutes; Cooking time: 0 minutes;
Nutritional Info: 265 Cal; 24 g Fats; 3.8 g Protein; 11.6 g Carb; 6.4 g Fiber;

Ingredients

- 4 slices of onion
- ½ of avocado, peeled, pitted, sliced
- 4 ounces arugula
- 1 orange, zested, peeled, sliced
- 1 teaspoon agave syrup

Extra:

- 1/8 teaspoon salt
- 1/8 teaspoon cayenne pepper
- 2 tablespoons key lime juice
- 2 tablespoons olive oil

Directions

1. Distribute avocado, oranges, onion, and arugula between two plates.
2. Mix together oil, salt, cayenne pepper, agave syrup and lime juice in a small bowl and then stir until mixed.
3. Drizzle the dressing over the salad and then serve.

Storage instructions:

Divide the salad evenly between two meal containers, cover with a lid, and then store the containers in the refrigerator for up to 5 days.

Dinner – Vegetable Soup

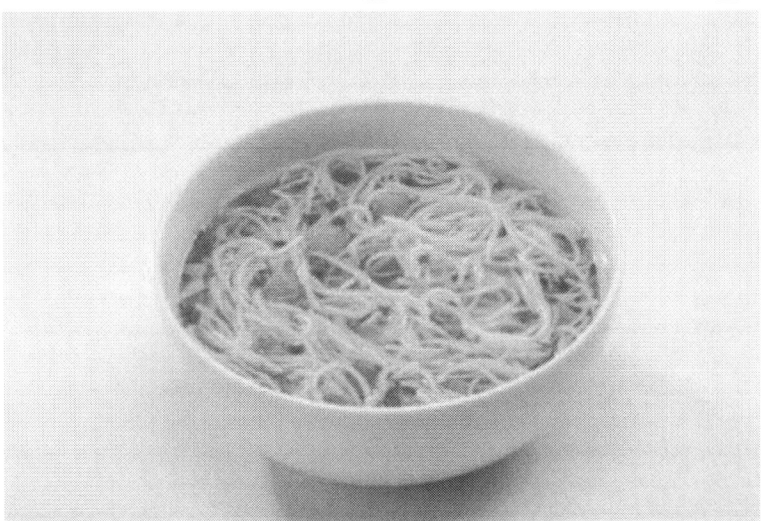

Serving: 2; Preparation time: 5 minutes; Cooking time: 12 minutes;

Nutritional Info: 265 Cal; 2 g Fats; 4 g Protein; 57 g Carb; 13.6 g Fiber;

Ingredients

- ½ of onion, peeled, cubed
- ½ of green bell pepper, chopped
- ½ of zucchini, grated
- 4 ounces sliced mushrooms, chopped
- ½ cup cherry tomatoes
- ¼ cup basil leaves
- 1 pack of spelt noodles, cooked
- ¼ teaspoon salt; 1/8 teaspoon cayenne pepper
- ½ of key lime, juiced
- 1 tablespoon grapeseed oil
- 2 cups spring water

Directions

1. Take a medium saucepan, place it over medium heat, add oil and when hot, add onion and then cook for 3 minutes or more until tender.
2. Add cherry tomatoes, bell pepper, and mushrooms, stir until mixed, and then continue cooking for 3 minutes until soft.
3. Add grated zucchini, season with salt, cayenne pepper, pour in the water, and then bring the mixture to a boil.
4. Then switch heat to the low level, add cooked noodles and then simmer the soup for 5 minutes. When done, ladle soup into two bowls, top with basil leaves, drizzle with lime juice and then serve.

Storage instructions:

Cool the soup, divide evenly between two meal prep containers, cover with a lid, and then store the containers in the refrigerator for up to 7 days.

Reheating instructions:

When ready to eat, reheat in the oven for 1 to 2 minutes until hot and then serve.

Day 3
Breakfast – Cantaloupe Smoothie

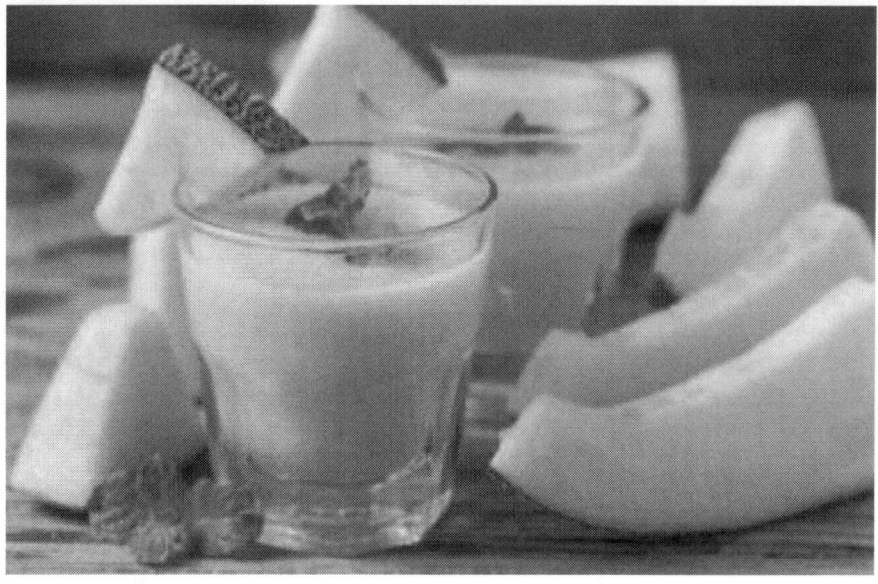

Serving: 2

Preparation time: 5 minutes; Cooking time: 0 minutes;
Nutritional Info: 114.7 Cal; 0.6 g Fats; 1.8 g Protein; 27.8 g Carb; 1 g Fiber;

Ingredients

- 1 cantaloupe, peeled, deseeded, sliced
- ½ cup Dr. Sebi Herbal Tea
- ½ of burro banana, peeled
- ½ cup soft-jelly coconut water

Directions

1. Plug in a high-speed food processor or blender and add all the ingredients in its jar.
2. Cover the blender jar with its lid and then pulse for 40 to 60 seconds until smooth.
3. Divide the drink between two glasses and then serve.

Storage instructions:

Divide drink between two jars or bottles, cover with a lid and then store the containers in the refrigerator for up to 3 days.

Lunch – Watermelon Refresher

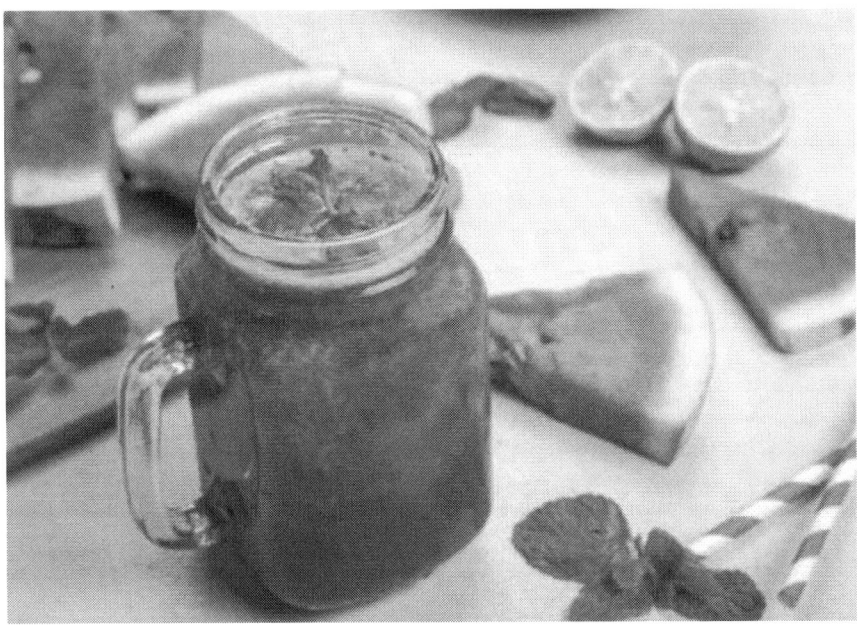

Serving: 2

Preparation time: 5 minutes; Cooking time: 0 minutes;
Nutritional Info: 55 Cal; 1.3 g Fats; 0.9 g Protein; 9.9 g Carb; 7 g Fiber;

Ingredients

- 1 watermelon, peeled, deseeded, cubed
- 1 tablespoon date sugar
- ½ of key lime, juiced, zest
- 2 cups soft-jelly coconut water

Directions

1. Place watermelon pieces in a high-speed food processor or blender, add lime zest and juice, add date sugar and then pulse until smooth.
2. Take two tall glasses, fill them with watermelon mixture until two-third full, and then pour in coconut water.
3. Stir until mixed and then serve.

Storage instructions:

Divide drink between two jars or bottles, cover with a lid and then store the containers in the refrigerator for up to 3 days.

Dinner – Cucumber and Basil Gazpacho

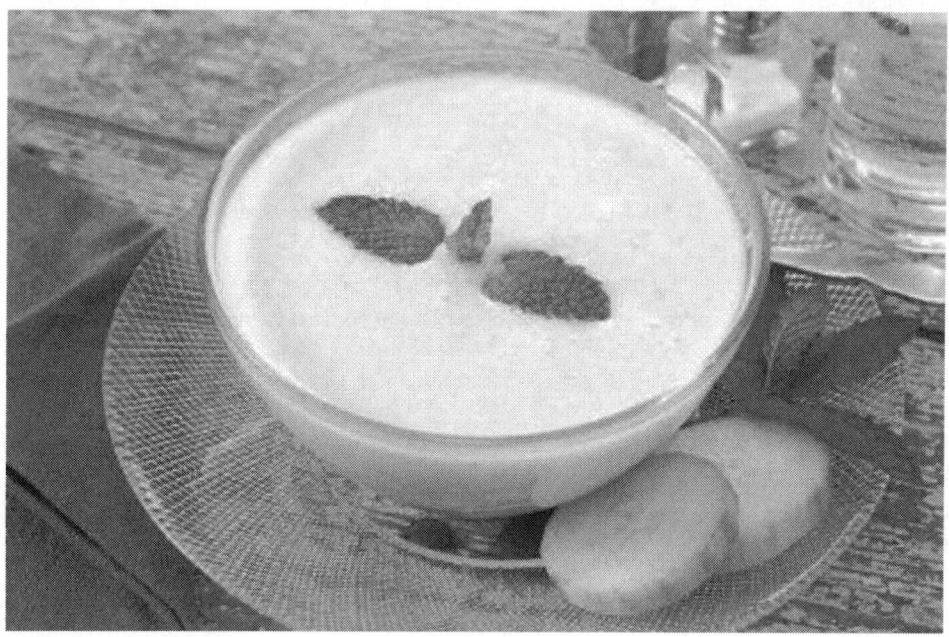

Serving: 2

Preparation time: 5 minutes; Cooking time: 0 minutes;
Nutritional Info: 190 Cal; 15 g Fats; 4 g Protein; 15 g Carb; 6 g Fiber;

Ingredients

- 1 avocado, peeled, pitted, cold
- 1 cucumber, deseeded, unpeeled, cold
- ½ cup basil leaves, cold
- ½ of key lime, juiced
- 2 cups spring water, chilled

Extra:

- 1 ½ teaspoon sea salt

Directions

1. Place all the ingredients into the jar of a high-speed food processor or blender and then pulse until smooth.
2. Tip the soup into a medium bowl and then chill for a minimum of 1 hour.
3. Divide the soup evenly between two bowls, top with some more basil and then serve.

Storage instructions:

Divide the gazpacho evenly between two meal prep containers, cover with a lid, and then store the containers in the refrigerator for up to 7 days.

Day 4
Breakfast – Kamut Porridge

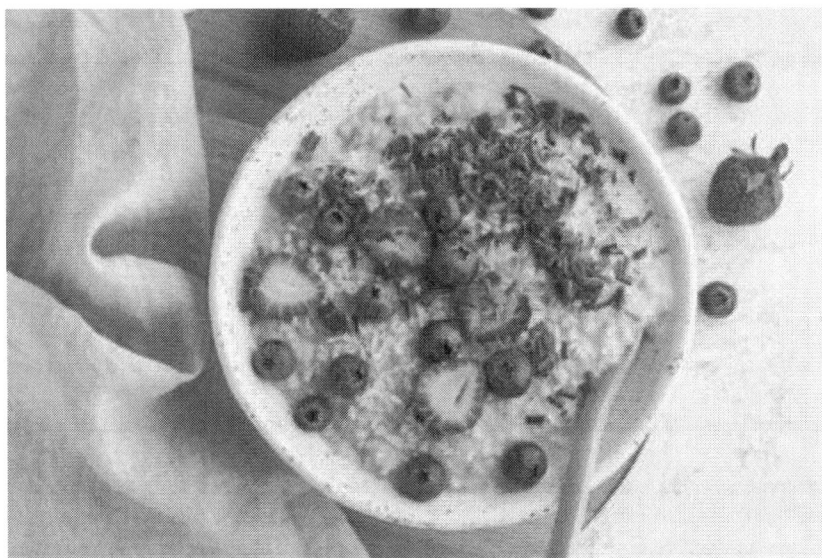

Serving: 2; **Preparation time: 5 minutes; Cooking time: 10 minutes;**

Nutritional Info: 183 Cal; 2 g Fats; 10 g Protein; 30 g Carb; 4 g Fiber;

Ingredients

- ½ cup Kamut
- ¼ teaspoon salt
- 2 tablespoons agave syrup
- ½ tablespoon coconut oil
- 2 cups walnut milk, homemade

Directions

1. Plug in a high-speed food processor or blender, add Kamut in its jar, and then pulse until cracked.
2. Take a medium saucepan, add Kamut in it along with salt, pour in the milk and then stir until combined.
3. Place the pan over high heat, bring the mixture to boil, then switch heat to medium-low level and simmer for 5 to 10 minutes until thickened to the desired level.
4. Then remove the pan from heat, stir agave syrup and oil into the porridge and then distribute evenly between two bowls.
5. Garnish the porridge with Dr. Sebi Diet's approved fruits and then serve.

Storage instructions:

Cool the porridge, divide evenly between two meal prep containers, cover with a lid, and then store the containers in the refrigerator for up to 7 days.

Reheating instructions:

When ready to eat, reheat in the oven for 1 to 2 minutes until hot and then serve with Dr. Sebi Diet's approved fruits.

Lunch – Zucchini Hummus Wrap

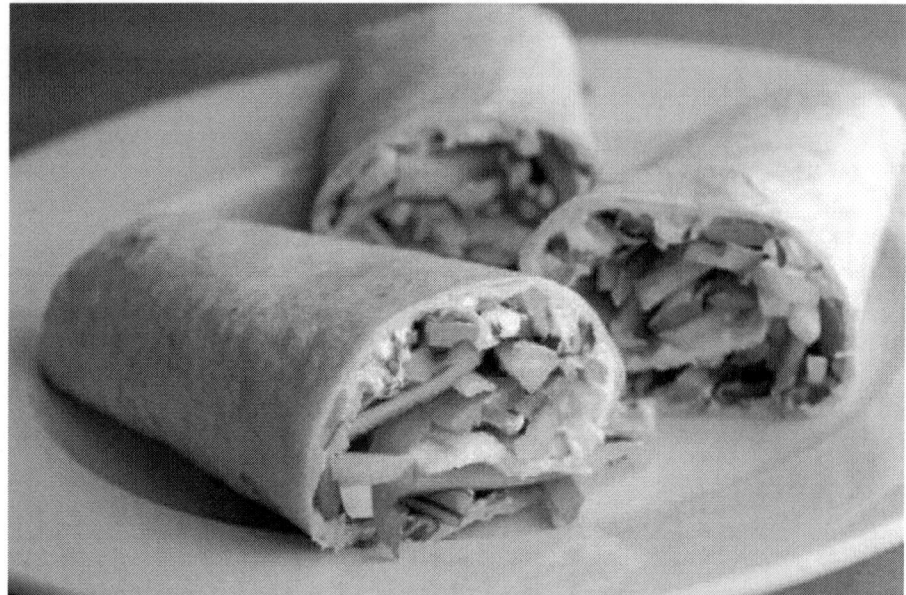

Serving: 2; **Preparation time: 10 minutes; Cooking time: 8 minutes;**

Nutritional Info: 264.5 Cal; 5.1 g Fats; 8.5 g Protein; 34.5 g Carb; 5 g Fiber;

Ingredients

- ½ cup iceberg lettuce
- 1 zucchini, sliced
- 2 cherry tomatoes, sliced
- 2 spelt flour tortillas
- 4 tablespoons homemade hummus
- ¼ teaspoon salt; 1/8 teaspoon cayenne pepper
- 1 tablespoon grapeseed oil

Directions

1. Take a grill pan, grease it oil and let it preheat over medium-high heat setting.
2. Meanwhile, place zucchini slices in a large bowl, sprinkle with salt and cayenne pepper, drizzle with oil and then toss until coated.
3. Arrange zucchini slices on the grill pan and then cook for 2 to 3 minutes per side until developed grill marks.
4. Assemble tortillas and for this, heat the tortilla on the grill pan until warm and develop grill marks and spread 2 tablespoons of hummus over each tortilla.
5. Distribute grilled zucchini slices over the tortillas, top with lettuce and tomato slices, and then wrap tightly.
6. Serve straight away.

Storage instructions:

Cover each wrap with a plastic wrap and foil and then refrigerate for up to 5 days.

Reheating instructions:

When ready to eat, bring the wrap to room temperature or reheat in the oven for 1 to 2 minutes until hot and then serve.

Dinner – Basil and Avocado Salad

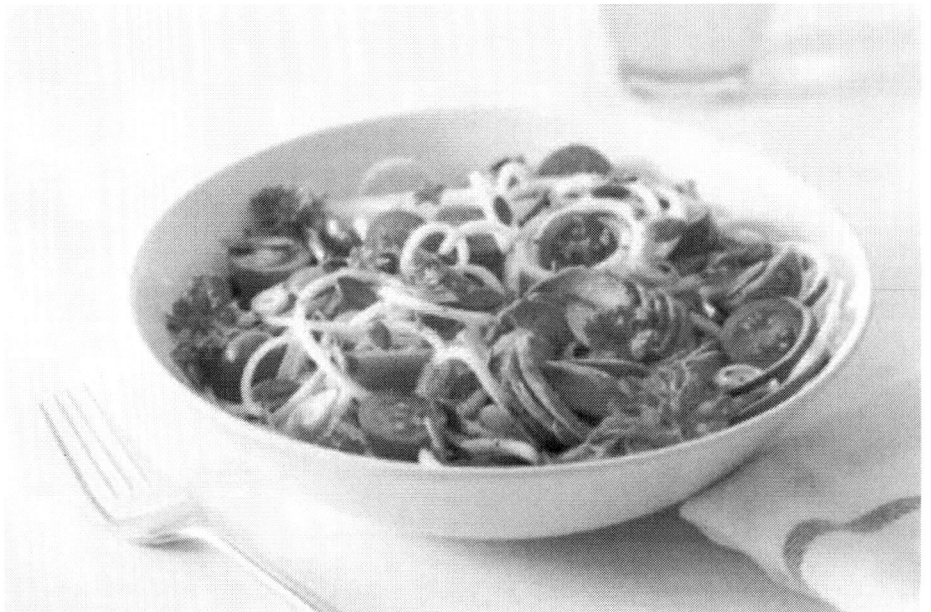

Serving: 2

Preparation time: 10 minutes; Cooking time: 0 minutes;
Nutritional Info: 387 Cal; 16.6 g Fats; 9.4 g Protein; 54.3 g Carb; 8.6 g Fiber;

Ingredients

- ½ cup avocado, peeled, pitted, chopped
- ½ cup basil leaves
- ½ cup cherry tomatoes
- 2 cups cooked spelt noodles

Extra:

- 1 teaspoon agave syrup
- 1 tablespoon key lime juice
- 2 tablespoons olive oil

Directions

1. Take a large bowl, place pasta in it, add tomato, avocado, and basil in it and then stir until mixed.
2. Take a small bowl, add agave syrup and salt in it, pour in lime juice and olive oil, and then whisk until combined.
3. Pour lime juice mixture over pasta, toss until combined, and then serve.

Storage instructions:

Divide the salad evenly between two meal prep containers, cover with a lid, and then store the containers in the refrigerator for up to 5 days.

Day 5
Breakfast – Smoothie Bowl

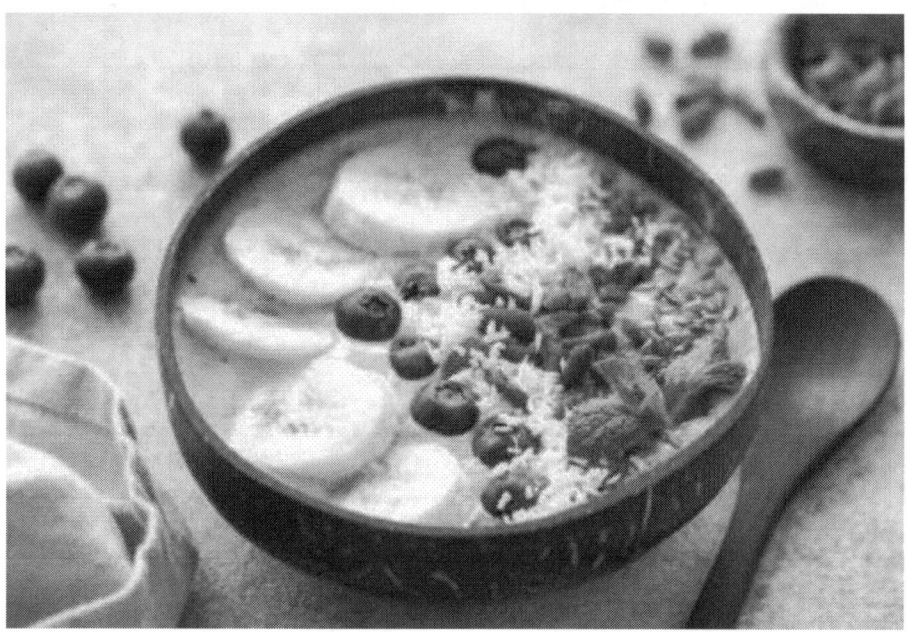

Serving: 2

Preparation time: 5 minutes; Cooking time: 0 minutes;
Nutritional Info: 338 Cal; 9.6 g Fats; 8.6 g Protein; 64.3 g Carb; 12.1 g Fiber;

Ingredients

- 1 burro banana, peeled
- 1 ½ cup mixed berries
- 1 mango, peeled, destoned, chopped
- 2 tablespoons walnut milk, homemade
- 1 tablespoon walnut butter, homemade

Extra:

- 2 tablespoons agave syrup

Directions

1. Plug in a high-speed food processor or blender, add banana and berries, and then pulse at low speed until small pieces of fruits remain in the jar.
2. Add milk, butter, and agave syrup, pulse until combined, and then divide the mixture evenly between two bowls.
3. Top evenly with mango slices and some more berries and then serve.

Storage instructions:

Divide drink between two jars or bottles, cover with a lid and then store the containers in the refrigerator for up to 3 days.

Lunch – Zucchini Bread Pancakes

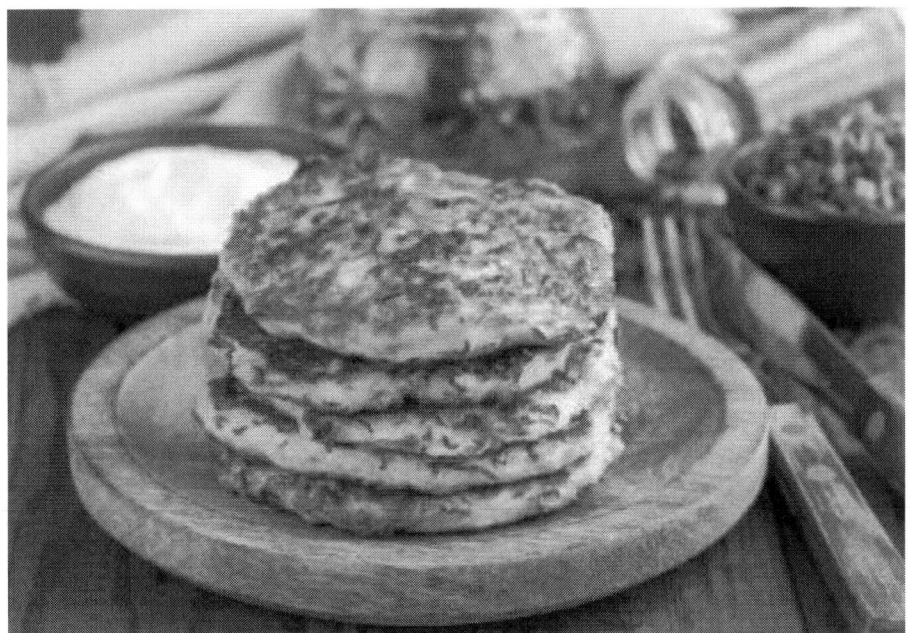

Serving: 2

Preparation time: 10 minutes; Cooking time: 8 minutes;
Nutritional Info: 130 Cal; 4 g Fats; 3 g Protein; 21 g Carb; 3 g Fiber;

Ingredients

- 1 cup spelt flour
- ½ cup grated zucchini
- ¼ cup chopped walnuts
- 1 cup walnut milk, homemade

Extra:
- 1 tablespoon date sugar
- 1 tablespoon grapeseed oil

Directions

1. Take a medium bowl, place flour in it, add date sugar, and then stir until mixed.
2. Add mashed banana and milk in it, whisk until smooth batter comes together, and then fold in nuts and zucchini until just mixed.
3. Take a large skillet, place over medium-high heat, add oil and when hot, pour the batter in it in portion and then shape each portion into a pancake.
4. Cook each pancake for 3 to 4 minutes per side and then serve.

Storage instructions:

Cool the pancakes, divide evenly between two meal prep containers, cover with a lid, and then store the containers in the refrigerator for up to 7 days.

Storage instructions:

When ready to eat, reheat in the oven for 1 to 2 minutes until hot and then serve.

Dinner – Dandelion and Strawberry Salad

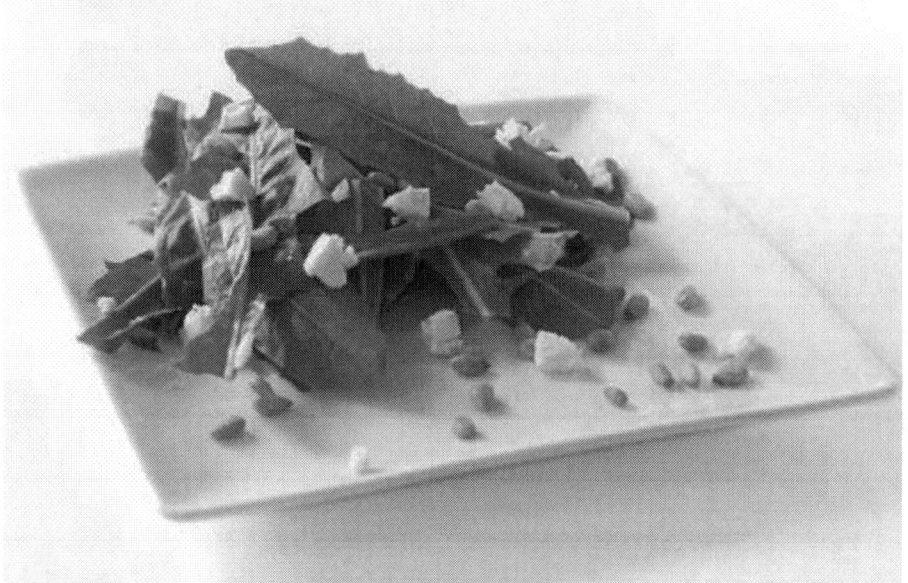

Serving: 2; **Preparation time: 10 minutes; Cooking time: 7 minutes;**

Nutritional Info: 204 Cal; 16.1 g Fats; 7 g Protein; 10.6 g Carb; 2.8 g Fiber;

Ingredients

- ½ of onion, peeled, sliced
- 5 strawberries, sliced
- 2 cups dandelion greens, rinsed
- 1 tablespoon key lime juice
- 1 tablespoon grapeseed oil
- ¼ teaspoon salt

Directions

1. Take a medium skillet pan, place it over medium heat, add oil and let it heat until warm.
2. Add onion, season with 1/8 teaspoon salt, stir until mixed, and then cook for 3 to 5 minutes until tender and golden brown.
3. Meanwhile, take a small bowl, place slices of strawberries in it, drizzle with ½ tablespoon lime juice and then toss until coated.
4. When onions have turned golden brown, stir in remaining lime juice, stir until mixed, and then cook for 1 minute.
5. Remove pan from heat, transfer onions into a large salad bowl, add strawberries along with their juices and dandelion greens and then sprinkle with remaining salt.
6. Toss until mixed and then serve.

Storage instructions:

Divide the salad evenly between two meal prep containers, cover with a lid, and then store the containers in the refrigerator for up to 5 days.

Day 6
Breakfast – Refreshing Smoothie with Nuts

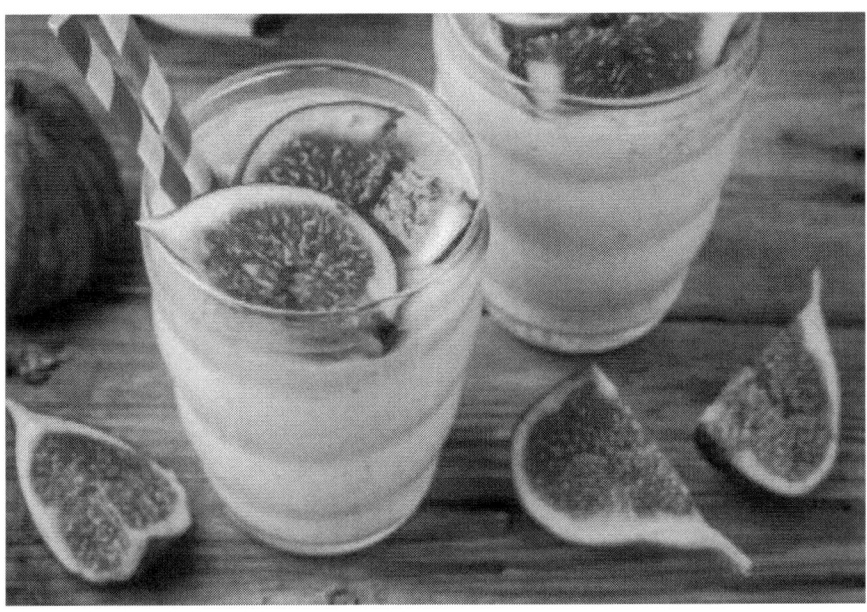

Serving: 2

Preparation time: 5 minutes; Cooking time: 0 minutes;
Nutritional Info: 234 Cal; 2 g Fats; 6.1 g Protein; 53.1 g Carb; 5.8 g Fiber;

Ingredients

- ½ of burro banana, peeled
- ½ cup figs
- 2 strawberries
- ¼ cup Brazil nuts
- 1 cup spring water

Directions

1. Plug in a high-speed food processor or blender and add all the ingredients in its jar.
2. Cover the blender jar with its lid and then pulse for 40 to 60 seconds until smooth.
3. Divide the drink between two glasses and then serve.

Storage instructions:

Divide drink between two jars or bottles, cover with a lid and then store the containers in the refrigerator for up to 3 days.

Lunch – Wakame Salad

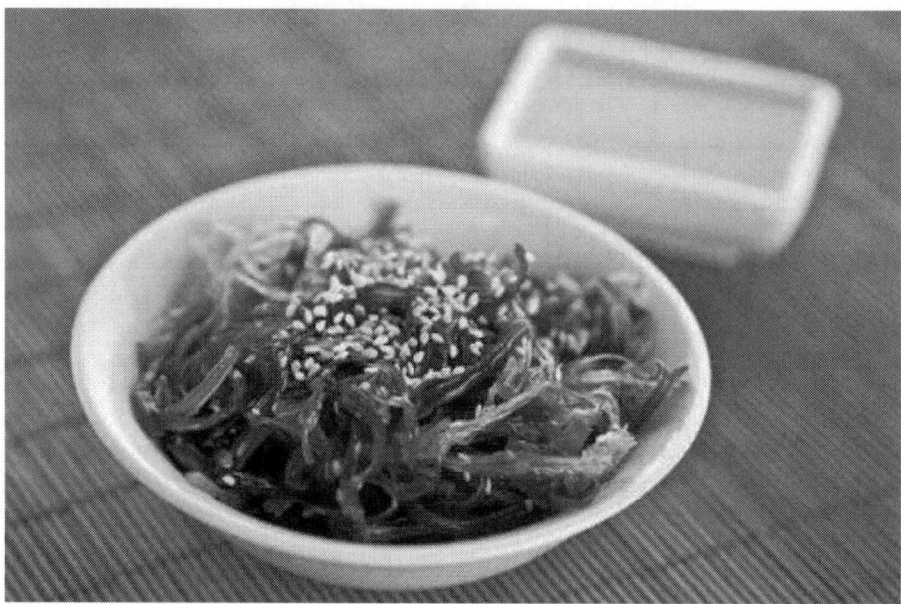

Serving: 2

Preparation time: 15 minutes; Cooking time: 0 minutes;
Nutritional Info: 106 Cal; 7.3 g Fats; 3 g Protein; 8 g Carb; 1.7 g Fiber;

Ingredients

- 1 cup wakame stems
- ½ tablespoon chopped red bell pepper
- ½ teaspoon onion powder
- ½ tablespoon key lime juice
- ½ teaspoon ginger powder

Extra:

- ½ tablespoon agave syrup
- ½ tablespoon sesame seeds
- ½ tablespoon sesame oil

Directions

1. Place wakame stems in a bowl, cover with water, let them soak for 10 minutes, and then drain.
2. Meanwhile, prepare the dressing and for this, take a small bowl, add lime juice, onion and ginger powder, agave syrup and sesame oil in it and then whisk until blended.
3. Place drained wakame stems in a large dish, add bell pepper, pour in the dressing and then toss until coated.
4. Sprinkle sesame seeds over the salad and then serve.

Storage instructions:

Divide the salad evenly between two meal prep containers, cover with a lid, and then store the containers in the refrigerator for up to 5 days.

Dinner – Portobello Burgers

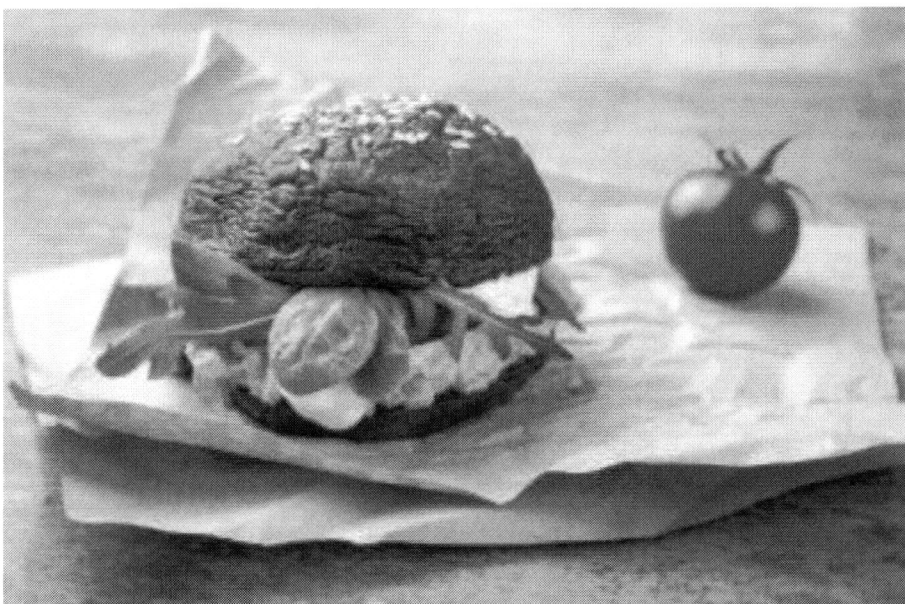

Serving: 2; **Preparation time: 10 minutes; Cooking time: 20 minutes;**

Nutritional Info: 354 Cal; 32.8 g Fats; 3.7 g Protein; 14.4 g Carb; 4.4 g Fiber;

Ingredients

- 2 Portobello mushroom caps
- ½ of avocado, sliced
- 1 cup purslane
- 2 teaspoons dried basil
- 2 tablespoons olive oil
- ¼ teaspoon salt; 1 teaspoon dried oregano
- ½ teaspoon cayenne pepper

Directions

1. Switch on the oven, then set it to 425 degrees F and let it preheat.
2. Prepare the marinade and for this, take a small bowl, pour in oil, add cayenne pepper, onion powder, oregano, and basil and then stir until mixed.
3. Take a cookie sheet, line it with a foil, brush with oil, place mushroom caps on it, evenly pour the marinade over mushroom caps and then let them marinate for 10 minutes.
4. Then bake the mushroom caps for 20 minutes, flipping halfway, until tender and cooked. When done, place mushroom caps on two plates, top the caps with avocado and purslane evenly.

Storage instructions:

Cool the mushroom caps, cover them in a plastic wrap and foil, and then store the containers in the refrigerator for up to 7 days.

Reheating instructions:

When ready to eat, reheat in the oven for 1 to 2 minutes until hot, top the caps with avocado and purslane evenly and then serve.

Day 7
Breakfast – Green Pancakes

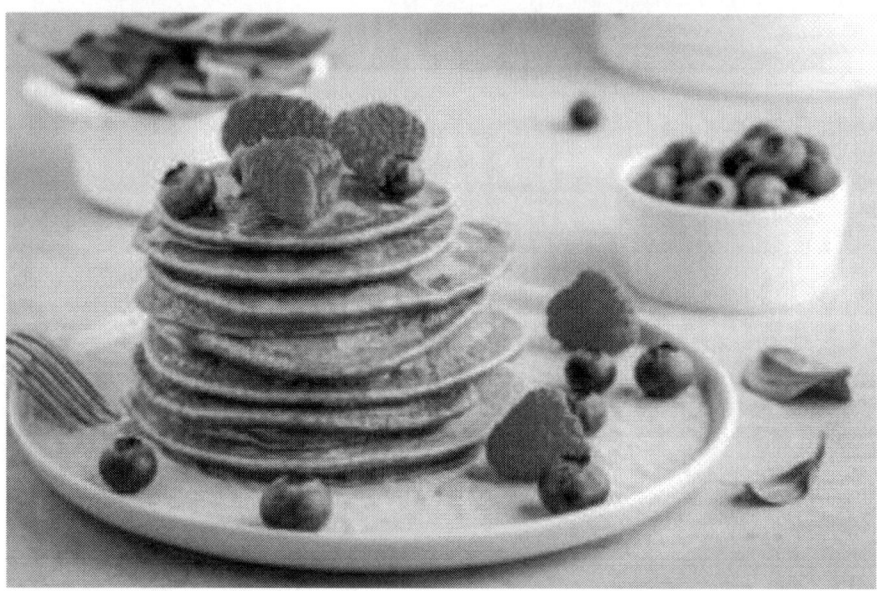

Serving: 2; Preparation time: 10 minutes; Cooking time: 6 minutes;

Nutritional Info: 144 Cal; 0.6 g Fats; 6 g Protein; 31.6 g Carb; 5.4 g Fiber;

Ingredients

- ½ cup chickpea flour
- ¼ cup blueberries
- 1 burro banana, peeled
- ½ cup amaranth greens
- ½ cup spring water; ½ teaspoon of sea salt
- 1 tablespoon agave syrup
- 1 tablespoon walnut butter
- 1 tablespoon grapeseed oil

Directions

1. Plug in a high-speed food processor or blender and add all the ingredients in its jar.
2. Cover the blender jar with its lid, pulse for 40 to 60 seconds until smooth, tip the mixture in a bowl and let it rest for 10 minutes.
3. When ready to cook, take a large frying pan, place it over medium-high heat, add oil and then let it heat.
4. Scoop prepared batter into the hot pan into six portions, shape each portion like a pancake and then cook for 2 to 3 minutes per side until edges have cooked and firm.

Storage instructions:

Cool the pancakes, divide evenly between two meal prep containers, cover with a lid, and then store the containers in the refrigerator for up to 7 days.

Reheating instructions:

When ready to eat, reheat in the oven for 1 to 2 minutes until hot and then serve.

Lunch – Grilled Romaine Lettuce Salad

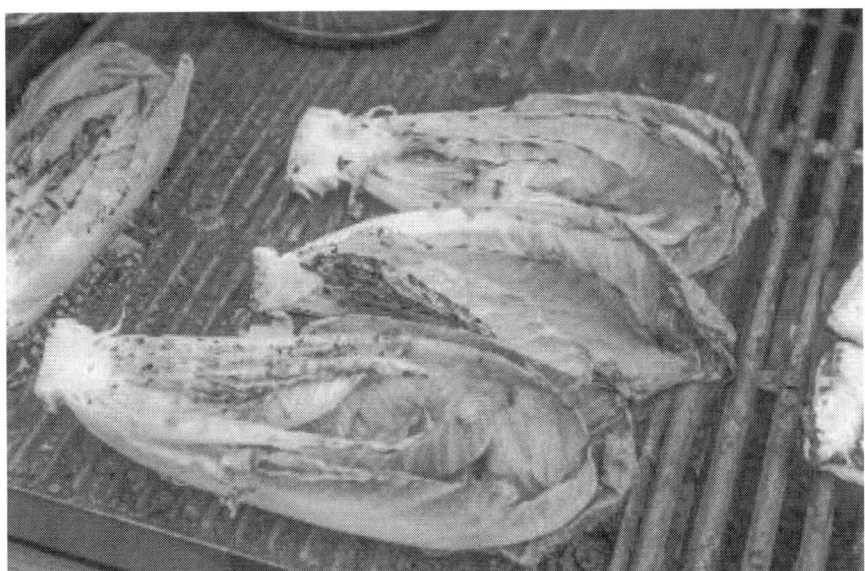

Serving: 2; **Preparation time: 10 minutes; Cooking time: 10 minutes;**

Nutritional Info: 130 Cal; 2 g Fats; 2 g Protein; 24 g Carb; 4 g Fiber;

Ingredients

- 2 small heads of romaine lettuce, cut in half
- 1 tablespoon chopped basil
- 1 tablespoon chopped red onion
- ¼ teaspoon onion powder
- ½ tablespoon agave syrup
- ½ teaspoon salt; ¼ teaspoon cayenne pepper
- 2 tablespoons olive oil
- 1 tablespoon key lime juice

Directions

1. Take a large skillet pan, place it over medium heat and when warmed, arrange lettuce heads in it, cut-side down, and then cook for 4 to 5 minutes per side until golden brown on both sides.
2. When done, transfer lettuce heads to a plate and then let them cool for 5 minutes.
3. Meanwhile, prepare the dressing and for this, place remaining ingredients in a small bowl and then stir until combined.
4. Drizzle the dressing over lettuce heads.

Storage instructions:

Cool the lettuce, divide evenly between two meal prep containers, cover with a lid, and then store the containers in the refrigerator for up to 7 days. Store the dressing in a mini meal prep container.

Reheating instructions:

When ready to eat, reheat in the microwave oven for 1 to 2 minutes until ho, drizzle with dressing and then serve.

Dinner – Vegetable Fajitas Tacos

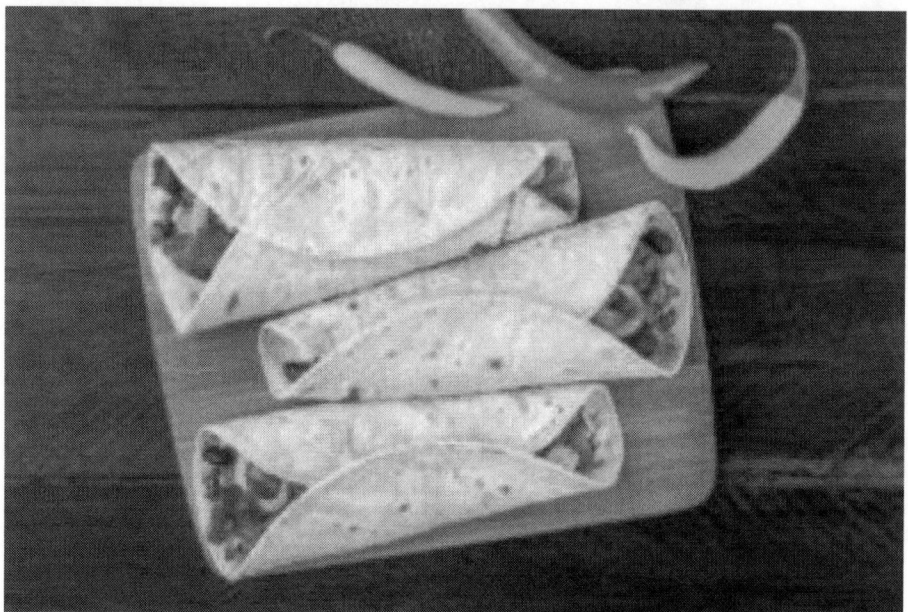

Serving: 2

Preparation time: 10 minutes; Cooking time: 8 minutes;
Nutritional Info: 337 Cal; 3.7 g Fats; 2.6 g Protein; 73.3 g Carb; 21.3 g Fiber;

Ingredients

- 2 Portobello mushroom caps, 1/3-inch sliced
- ¾ of red bell pepper, sliced
- ½ of onion, peeled, sliced
- ½ of key lime, juiced
- 2 spelt flour tortillas

Extra:

- 1/3 teaspoon salt; ¼ teaspoon cayenne pepper
- ¼ teaspoon onion powder
- 1 tablespoon grapeseed oil

Directions

1. Take a medium skillet pan, place it over medium heat, add oil and when hot, add onion and red pepper, and then cook for 2 minutes until tender-crisp.
2. Add mushrooms slices, sprinkle with all the seasoning, stir until mixed, and then cook for 5 minutes until vegetables turn soft.
3. Heat the tortilla until warm, distribute vegetables in their center, drizzle with lime juice, and then roll tightly.

Storage instructions:

Cool the wraps, cover with a plastic wrap and then with foil, and then store in the refrigerator for up to 5 days.

Reheating instructions:

When ready to eat, reheat in the oven for 1 to 2 minutes until hot and then serve.

Week 3

Shopping List

Shop for the following.

- Agave syrup
- Alkaline cherry tomato dressing
- Alkaline garlic sauce
- Apples, large
- Avocado, large
- Banana
- Basil
- Blueberries, 1 pint
- Bread crumbs
- Bromide Plus Powder
- Butternut squash, diced, 10 oz.
- Cayenne pepper
- Cherry tomatoes, 1 pint
- Chickpeas, 15.5 oz.
- Cilantro
- Cilantro, 1 bunch
- Coconut nectar
- Cucumber, large
- Date sugar
- Dried cherries
- Dried oregano
- Dried sage
- Dried thyme
- Fresh orange juice
- Grapeseed oil
- Grated / powdered ginger
- Green bell pepper, large
- Green leaf lettuce
- Ground cardamom
- Ground cinnamon
- Ground cloves
- Ground nutmeg
- Ground turmeric
- Homemade walnut milk
- Kale, bunch
- Kamut flakes
- Key limes
- Linseed
- Mango, large
- Medjool date
- Minced / powdered garlic
- Olive oil
- Olives, pitted, 6 oz.
- Onion powder
- Orange, large
- Parsley
- Pear, large
- Pumpkin seeds
- Red bell pepper, large
- Red onion, large
- Sea Salt
- Sea moss gel
- Sliced mushrooms, 8 oz.
- Soft-jelly coconut milk
- Soft-jelly coconut water
- Spelt burgers
- Spelt pasta
- Spring water
- Tri-color quinoa
- Turnip greens
- Vanilla extract
- Walnut butter
- Walnuts
- Watercress, 1 bunch
- Wild rice, 16 oz.
- Zucchini, large

Day 1
Breakfast – Apple Baked

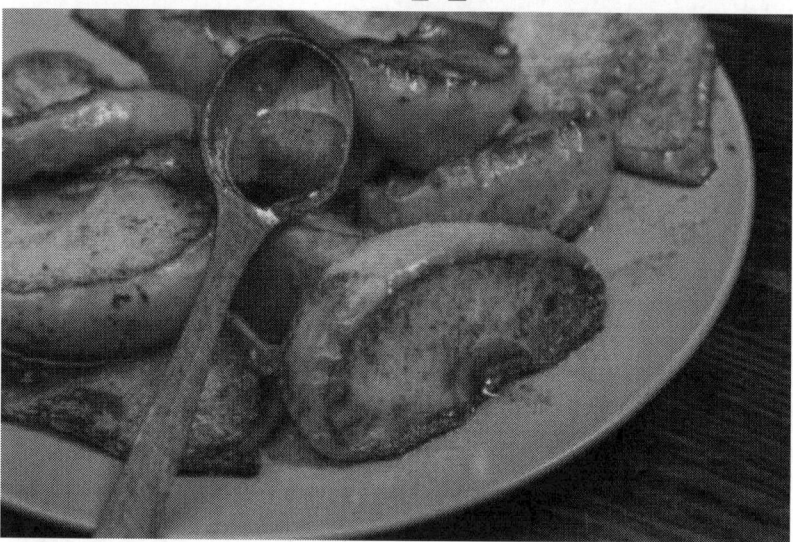

Serving: 2

Preparation time: 10 minutes; Cooking time: 55 minutes;
Nutritional Info: 346 Cal; 6.4 g Fats; 1.5 g Protein; 78 g Carb; 6.2 g Fiber;

Ingredients

- 4 apples, large, cored, sliced
- 1/8 teaspoon ground cloves
- 3 tablespoons agave syrup
- 1 tablespoon chopped walnuts

Directions

1. Switch on the oven, then set it to 350 degrees F and let it preheat.
2. Meanwhile, take a large bowl, place apple slices in it, drizzle with agave syrup and then toss until evenly coated.
3. Take a small bowl, place nuts in it, add cloves, and then stir until mixed.
4. Sprinkle nuts mixture over the apple and let it rest for 5 minutes or more until apples start releasing their juices.
5. Take a medium casserole dish, arrange apple slices on it, and then bake for 15 minutes.
6. Cover the casserole dish with foil and then continue baking for 40 minutes until bubbly.

Storage instructions:

Cool the apples, divide evenly between two containers, cover with a lid, and then store the containers in the refrigerator for up to 7 days.

Reheating instructions:

When ready to eat, reheat in the oven for 1 to 2 minutes until hot and then serve.

Lunch – Orange and Avocado Salad

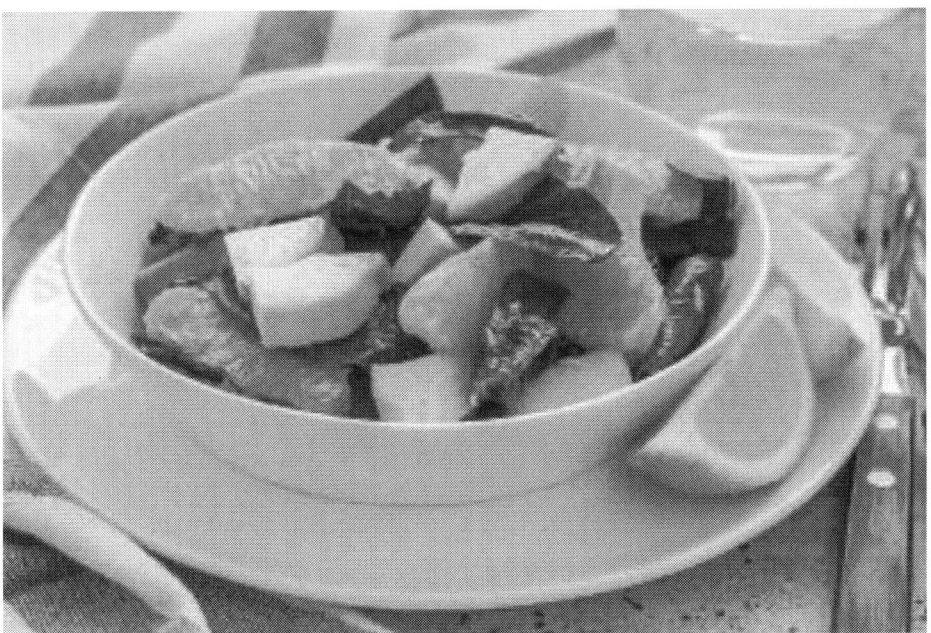

Serving: 2

Preparation time: 5 minutes; Cooking time: 0 minutes;
Nutritional Info: 228 Cal; 18.9 g Fats; 3.3 g Protein; 14.7 g Carb; 7 g Fiber;

Ingredients

- 1 orange, peeled, sliced
- 4 cups greens
- ½ of avocado, peeled, pitted, diced
- 2 tablespoons slivered red onion
- ½ cup cilantro

Extra:

- ¼ teaspoon salt
- ¼ cup olive oil
- 2 tablespoons lime juice
- 2 tablespoons orange juice

Directions

1. Prepare the dressing and for this, place cilantro in a food processor, pour in orange juice, lime juice, and oil, add salt and then pulse until blended.
2. Tip the dressing into a salad bowl, add remaining ingredients, toss until coated.

Storage instructions:

Divide the salad evenly between two containers, cover with a lid, and then store the containers in the refrigerator for up to 5 days.

Dinner – Chickpea Loaf

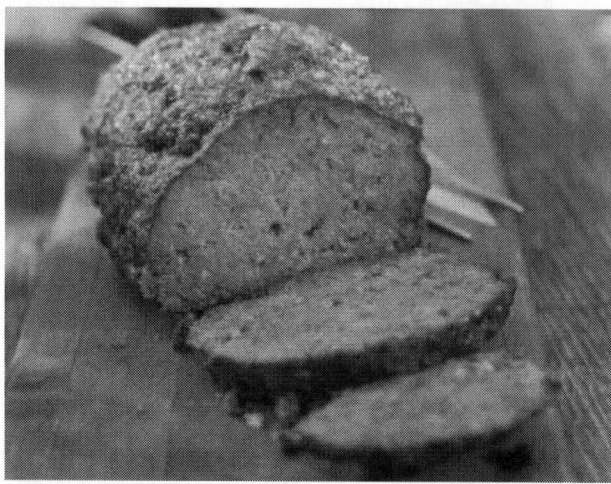

Serving: 2; **Preparation time: 10 minutes; Cooking time: 45 minutes;**

Nutritional Info: 268.7 Cal; 6.2 g Fats; 10.3 g Protein; 46 g Carb; 9.4 g Fiber;

Ingredients

- ¼ cup spelt flour
- 1 ½ cups chickpeas, cooked
- ¾ cup diced onions
- ¼ cup minced basil
- ½ cup sliced white mushrooms
- 1 red bell pepper, cored, diced
- 1 tablespoon grapeseed oil
- 1 tablespoon and ¼ teaspoon granulated onion, homemade
- 1/8 teaspoon dried thyme; ½ teaspoon sea salt and more as needed
- 1/3 teaspoon dried sage; ¼ teaspoon cayenne pepper and more as needed
- ¼ teaspoon dried oregano

Directions

1. Switch on the oven, then set it to 350 degrees F and let it preheat.
2. Meanwhile, take a large skillet pan, place it over medium-high heat, add oil in it and when hot, add onion, pepper, and mushroom and then cook for 3 minutes or until begin to tender. Add minced basil into the pan, stir until mixed, remove the pan from heat, add all the seasonings and then stir until mixed.
3. Place chickpeas in a food processor, pulse until coarsely chopped, and then transfer into a medium bowl. Add cooked vegetable mixture along with remaining ingredients, stir until well mixed and then spoon into a greased loaf pan.
4. Bake the loaf for 30 to 40 minutes until firm and cooked, cool it slightly, cut into slices.

Storage instructions:

Cool the meatloaf slices, divide evenly between two containers, cover with a lid, and then store the containers in the refrigerator for up to 7 days.

Reheating instructions:

When ready to eat, reheat in the oven for 1 to 2 minutes until hot and then serve.

Day 2
Breakfast – Watercress Detox Smoothie

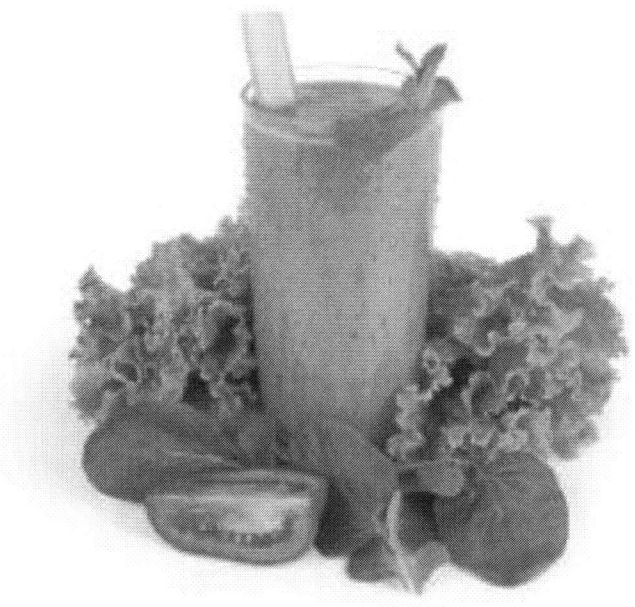

Serving: 2

Preparation time: 5 minutes; Cooking time: 0 minutes;
Nutritional Info: 146 Cal; 10.5 g Fats; 7 g Protein; 7.5 g Carb; 2.5 g Fiber;

Ingredients

- ½ cup watercress
- ½ of avocado, peeled, pitted
- 1 key lime, juiced
- 1 cup soft-jelly coconut milk, homemade
- 1 teaspoon Bromide Plus Powder

Directions

1. Plug in a high-speed food processor or blender and add all the ingredients in its jar.
2. Cover the blender jar with its lid and then pulse for 40 to 60 seconds until smooth.
3. Divide the drink between two glasses.

Storage instructions:

Divide drink between two jars or bottles, cover with a lid and then store the containers in the refrigerator for up to 3 days.

Lunch – Mix Veggie Mushroom Salad

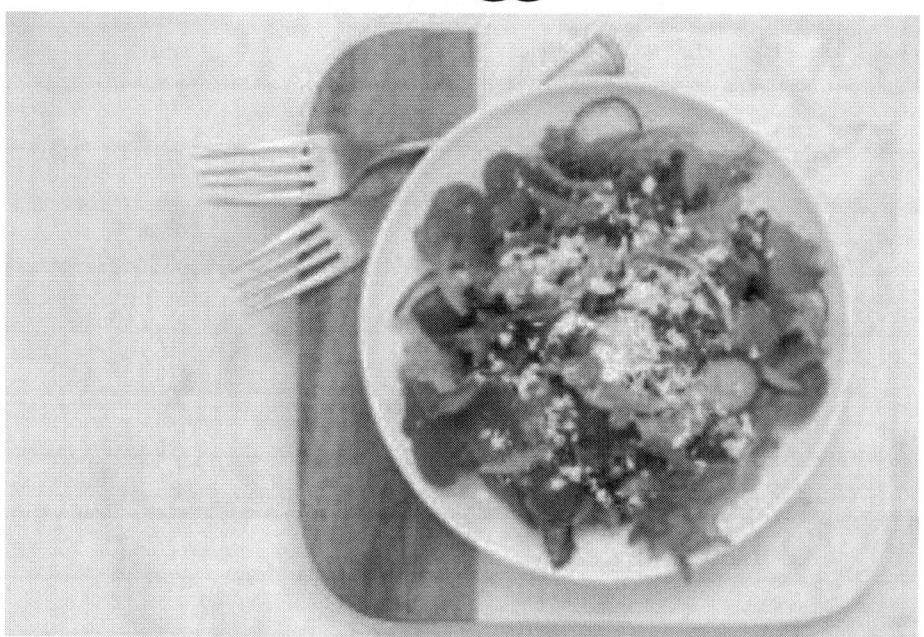

Serving: 2

Preparation time: 5 minutes; Cooking time: 0 minutes;
Nutritional Info: 129 Cal; 7 g Fats; 2 g Protein; 14 g Carb; 4 g Fiber;

Ingredients

- ½ of a medium cucumber, deseeded, chopped
- 6 leaves of lettuce, broke into pieces
- 4 mushrooms, chopped
- 6 cherry tomatoes, chopped
- 10 olives

Extra:

- ½ of lime, juiced
- 1 teaspoon olive oil
- ¼ teaspoon salt

Directions

1. Take a medium salad bowl, place all the ingredients in it and then toss until mixed.

Storage instructions:

Divide the salad evenly between two meal prep containers, cover with a lid, and then store the containers in the refrigerator for up to 5 days.

Dinner – Fried Rice

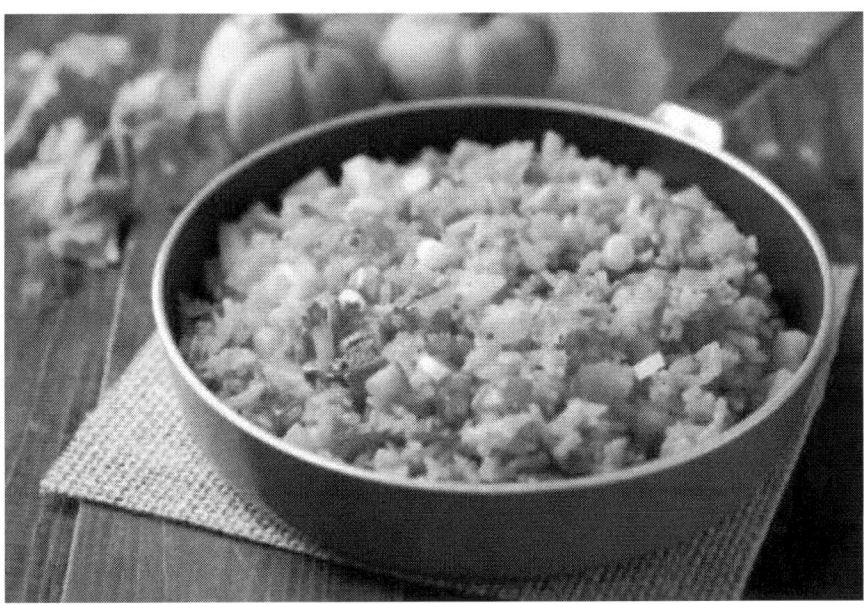

Serving: 2

Preparation time: 5 minutes; Cooking time: 15 minutes;
Nutritional Info: 140 Cal; 7 g Fats; 4 g Protein; 15 g Carb; 1.1 g Fiber;

Ingredients

- ½ cup sliced mushrooms
- 1 cup cooked wild rice
- ½ cup sliced red bell pepper
- ¼ of a medium onion, peeled, cubed
- ½ cup sliced zucchini

Extra:

- ½ teaspoon salt
- ¼ teaspoon cayenne pepper
- 1 tablespoon grapeseed oil

Directions

1. Take a medium skillet pan, place it over medium heat, add oil and when hot, add onion and cook for 5 minutes until browned.
2. Add remaining vegetables, stir until mixed, and then cook for 5 minutes until almost soft.
3. Add rice, stir until combined and cook for 3 minutes until golden brown.

Storage instructions:

Cool the rice, divide evenly between two meal containers, cover with a lid, and then store the containers in the refrigerator for up to 7 days.

Reheating instructions:

When ready to eat, reheat in the oven for 1 to 2 minutes until hot and then serve.

Day 3
Breakfast – Mango and Orange Smoothie

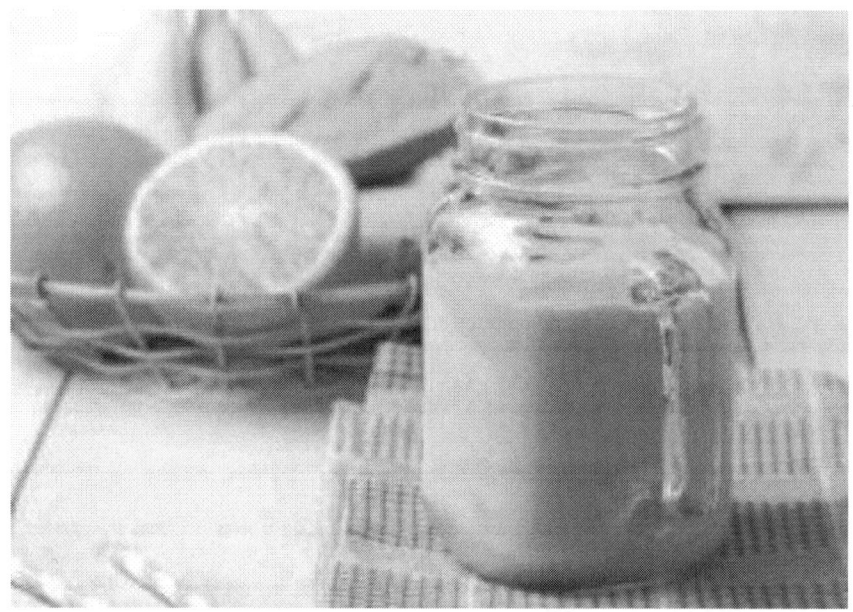

Serving: 2

Preparation time: 5 minutes; Cooking time: 0 minutes;
Nutritional Info: 163 Cal; 3.4 g Fats; 1 g Protein; 32 g Carb; 6 g Fiber;

Ingredients

- ½ of a large mango, peeled, destoned, cubed
- 1 key lime, juiced
- 1 orange, peeled
- 1 tablespoon agave syrup
- 1 tablespoon grapeseed oil

Extra:

- 1 cup herbal tea

Directions

1. Plug in a high-speed food processor or blender and add all the ingredients in its jar.
2. Cover the blender jar with its lid and then pulse for 40 to 60 seconds until smooth.
3. Divide the drink between two glasses.

Storage instructions:

Divide drink between two bottles or jars, cover with lids and then store the containers in the refrigerator for up to 3 days.

Lunch – Banana Fries

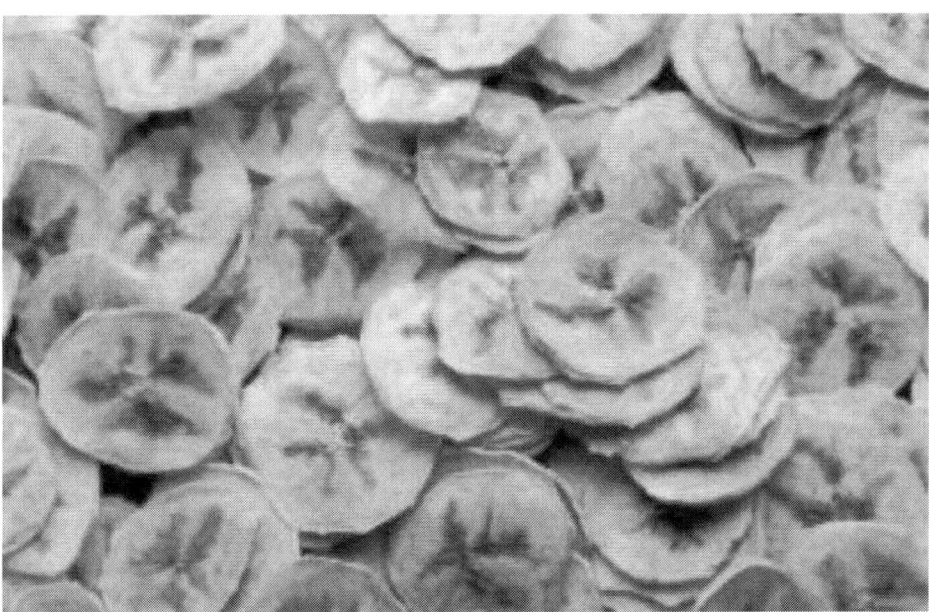

Serving: 2

Preparation time: 5 minutes; Cooking time: 10 minutes;
Nutritional Info: 130.5 Cal; 6.5 g Fats; 1 g Protein; 20 g Carb; 3 g Fiber;

Ingredients

- 4 baby burro bananas, peeled, cut in squares
- ¼ teaspoon salt
- ½ of a medium onion, peeled, chopped
- ½ of medium green bell pepper, cored, chopped
- 2 teaspoons grapeseed oil

Extra:

- ¼ teaspoon cayenne pepper

Directions

1. Take a medium pan, place over medium-low heat, add oil and when hot, add banana pieces and then cook for 3 minutes or until beginning to brown.
2. Then turn the banana pieces, add remaining ingredients, stir until mixed, and then continue cooking for 5 to 7 minutes until onions have caramelized.

Storage instructions:

Cool the chips, divide evenly between two containers, cover with a lid, and then store the containers in the refrigerator for up to 7 days.

Reheating instructions:

When ready to eat, reheat in the oven for 1 to 2 minutes until hot and then serve.

Dinner – Zoodles with Basil and Avocado Sauce

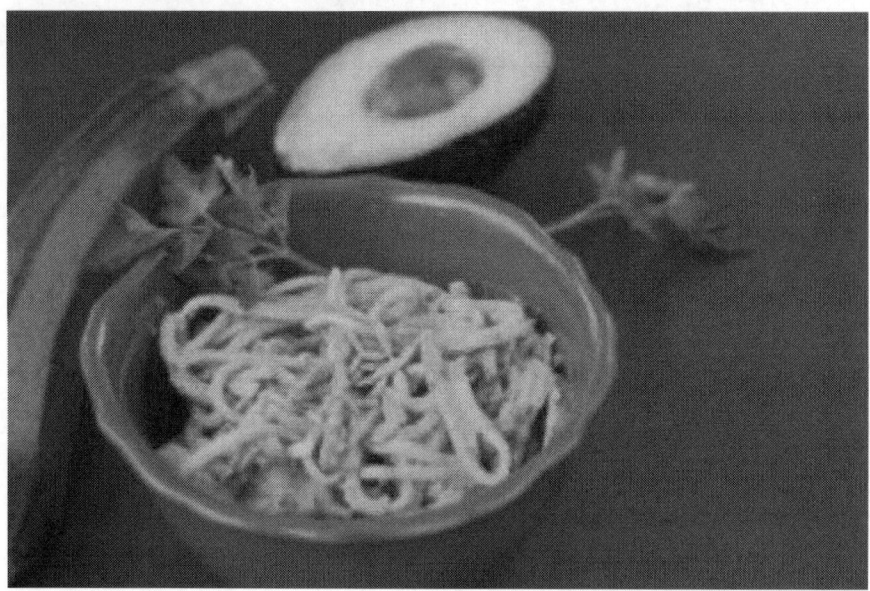

Serving: 2

Preparation time: 10 minutes; Cooking time: 0 minutes;
Nutritional Info: 330 Cal; 20.7 g Fats; 7.1 g Protein; 35.3 g Carb; 7.8 g Fiber;

Ingredients

- 2 zucchinis, spiralized into noodles
- 2 avocados, peeled, pitted
- ½ cup walnuts
- 2 cups basil leaves
- 24 cherry tomatoes, sliced

Extra:

- 1/3 teaspoon salt
- 4 tablespoons key lime juice
- ½ cup spring water

Directions

1. Prepare the sauce and for this, place all the ingredients except for zucchini noodles and tomatoes in a food processor and then pulse until smooth.
2. Take a large bowl, place zucchini noodles in it, add tomato slices, pour in the prepared sauce and then toss until coated.

Storage instructions:

Divide the noodles evenly between two containers, cover with a lid, and then store the containers in the refrigerator for up to 3 days.

Day 4
Breakfast – Green Smoothie with Apple and Blueberries

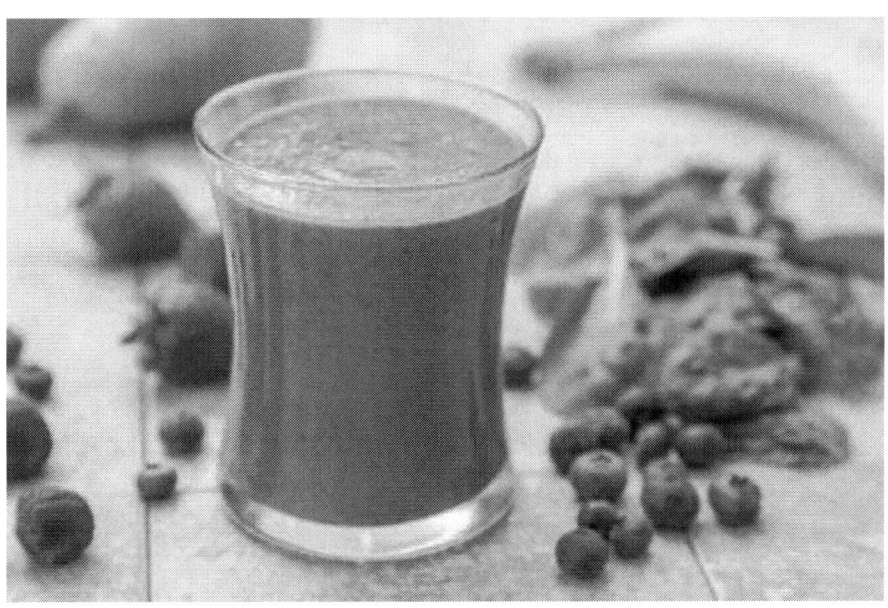

Serving: 2

Preparation time: 5 minutes; Cooking time: 0 minutes;
Nutritional Info: 215 Cal; 1.1 g Fats; 2.3 g Protein; 48 g Carb; 8.3 g Fiber;

Ingredients

- 1 cup blueberries
- 1 apple, cored
- 1 cup turnip greens
- ¼ cup Brazil nuts
- ½ tablespoon agave syrup

Extra:

- 1 cup walnut milk, homemade

Directions

1. Plug in a high-speed food processor or blender and add all the ingredients in its jar.
2. Cover the blender jar with its lid and then pulse for 40 to 60 seconds until smooth.
3. Divide the drink between two glasses.

Storage instructions:

Divide drink between two jars or bottles, cover with a lid and then store the containers in the refrigerator for up to 3 days.

Lunch – Sea Moss Smoothie

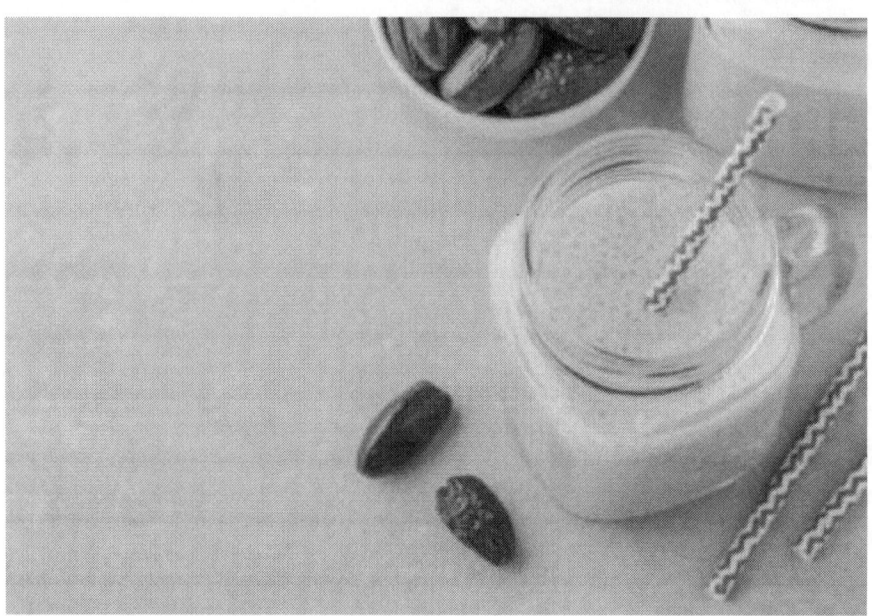

Serving: 2

Preparation time: 10 minutes; Cooking time: 0 minutes;
Nutritional Info: 100.5 Cal; 0.1 g Fats; 1.7 g Protein; 22.5 g Carb; 3.5 g Fiber;

Ingredients

- 33 g sea moss, rinsed
- 2/3 tablespoon linseed
- 1 tablespoon coconut nectar
- 2 cups spring water, warmed
- 1 cup walnut milk, unsweetened

Extra:

- 1/8 teaspoon ground nutmeg
- 1/8 teaspoon ground cinnamon
- 1 teaspoon vanilla extract, unsweetened

Directions

1. Place rinsed seaweed in a medium bowl, add linseed, pour in the water and let it soak for a minimum of 4 hours until thickened slightly.
2. Drain the soaked sea moss, transfer into a food processor, pulse until the smooth paste comes together, and then refrigerate until required.
3. When ready to drink, transfer 8 tablespoons of sea moss paste into a food processor, add remaining ingredients and then pulse until smooth.
4. Divide the drink evenly between two glasses.

Storage instructions:

Divide drink between two jars, cover with a lid and then store the containers in the refrigerator for up to 3 days.

Dinner – Kamut Porridge with Dates

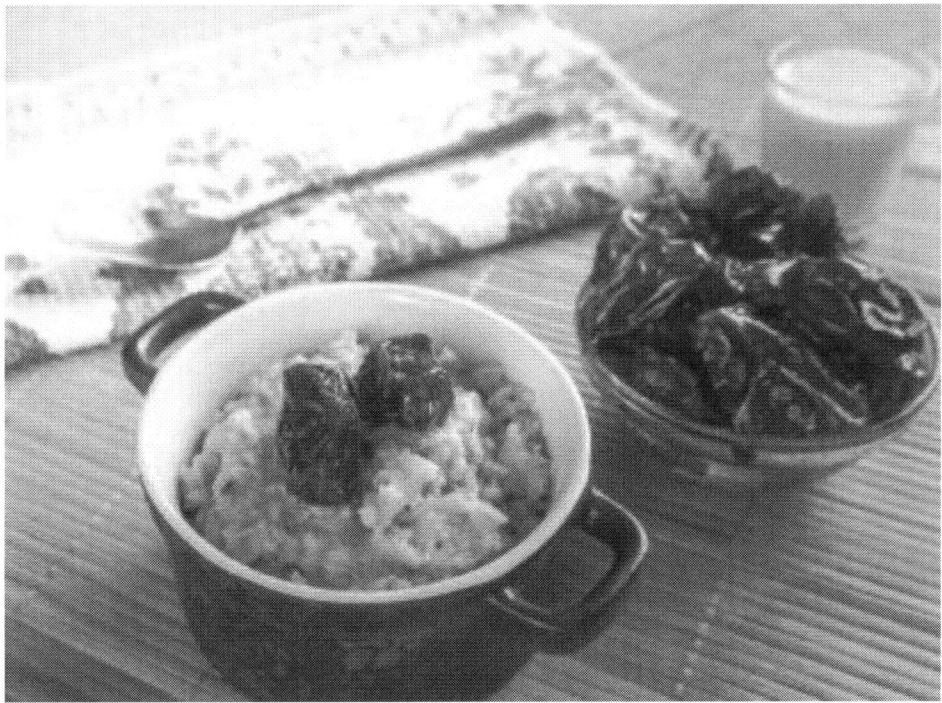

Serving: 2

Preparation time: 5 minutes; Cooking time: 15 minutes;

Nutritional Info: 132 Cal; 1 g Fats; 0.3 g Protein; 30.2 g Carb; 2 g Fiber;

Ingredients

- 1 cup Medjool dates, pitted, chopped
- 1 cup rolled Kamut flakes
- 1/8 teaspoon salt
- 1/16 teaspoon vanilla extract
- 2 cups spring water

Directions

4. Place Kamut flakes in a small saucepan, pour in the water, and let soak for overnight.
5. Then stir in salt, place the pan over medium-high heat and bring the mixture to a slow boil.
6. Switch heat to medium-low level and then continue cooking for 10 minutes or more until all the liquid has absorbed.
7. Remove pan from heat, add dates and vanilla into the porridge and then stir until mixed.
8. Divide porridge between two bowls, drizzle with agave syrup if needed.

Storage instructions:

Cool the porridge, divide evenly between two meal containers, cover with a lid, and then store the containers in the refrigerator for up to 7 days.

Reheating instructions:

When ready to eat, reheat in the oven for 1 to 2 minutes until hot, drizzle with agave syrup and then serve.

Day 5
Breakfast – Zucchini and Avocado Smoothie

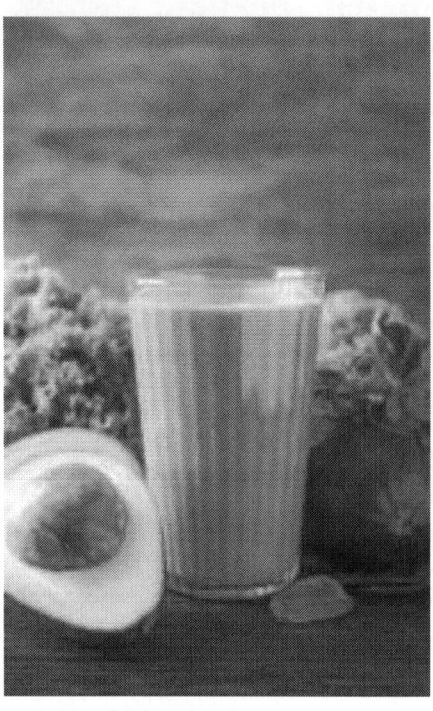

Serving: 2

Preparation time: 5 minutes; Cooking time: 0 minutes;
Nutritional Info: 165 Cal; 6.8 g Fats; 8.5 g Protein; 17.3 g Carb; 5.5 g Fiber;

Ingredients

- 3 tablespoons hemp seeds
- 1/3 cup diced zucchini
- 1 cup dandelion greens
- ¼ of a large avocado, peeled, pitted
- 1 ¼ cup walnut milk, homemade

Directions

1. Plug in a high-speed food processor or blender and add all the ingredients in its jar.
2. Cover the blender jar with its lid and then pulse for 40 to 60 seconds until smooth.
3. Divide the drink between two glasses.

Storage instructions:

Divide drink between two jars, cover with a lid and then store the containers in the refrigerator for up to 3 days.

Lunch – Kamut Pasta

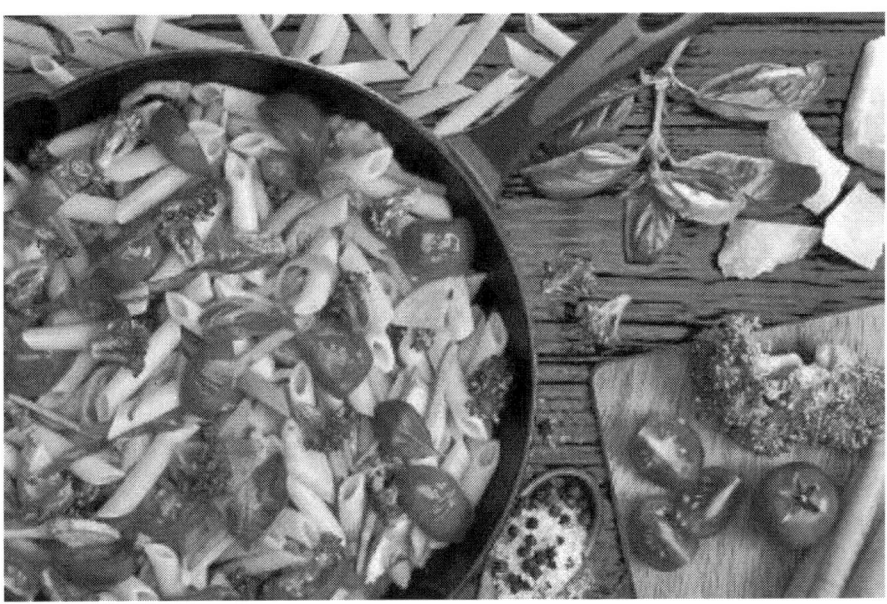

Serving: 2

Preparation time: 5 minutes; Cooking time: 0 minutes;
Nutritional Info: 143.7 Cal; 1.8 g Fats; 4.5 g Protein; 29.1 g Carb; 4.8 g Fiber;

Ingredients

- ½ cup sliced zucchini
- 2 cups cooked spelt pasta
- ¼ cup diced onions
- ½ cup diced green bell peppers
- ¼ cup cherry tomatoes, cut in half
  Extra:
- 2 tablespoons olives

Directions

1. Take a large bowl, place all the ingredients in it and then toss until well coated.

Storage instructions:

Cool the pasta, divide evenly between two meal containers, cover with a lid, and then store the containers in the refrigerator for up to 7 days.

Reheating instructions:

When ready to eat, reheat in the oven for 1 to 2 minutes until hot and then serve.

Dinner – Quinoa and Wild Rice

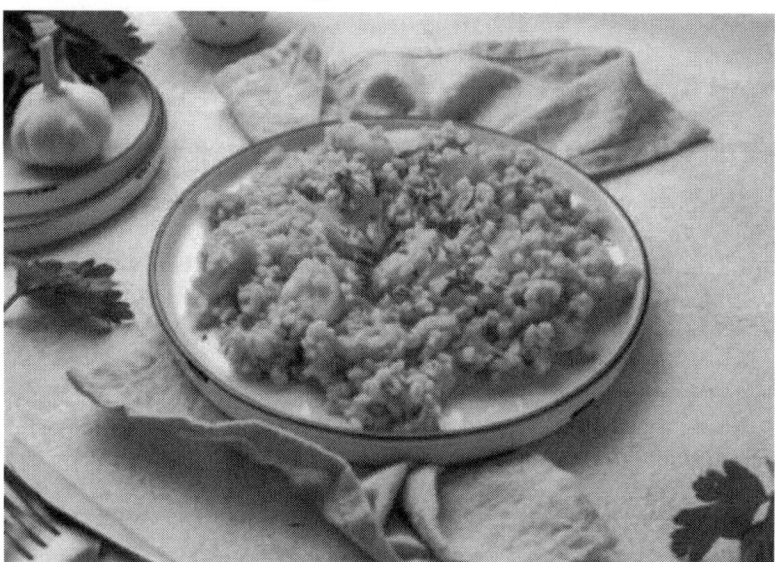

Serving: 2; **Preparation time: 10 minutes; Cooking time: 18 minutes;**

Nutritional Info: 132 Cal; 3.5 g Fats; 4.5 g Protein; 22 g Carb; 2 g Fiber;

Ingredients

- ½ cup wild rice, boiled
- 2 tablespoons dried cherries
- ½ cup tricolor quinoa, uncooked
- ½ key lime, zested
- ¼ cup cherry tomato dressing, homemade
- ½ teaspoon salt, divided; 1/8 teaspoon cayenne pepper
- 1/8 teaspoon ground cardamom
- ½ tablespoon olive oil
- ½ cup spring water

Directions

1. Cook the quinoa, and for this, take a medium saucepan, place it over medium heat, add oil and when hot, add quinoa and cook for 3 minutes until softened.
2. Pour in the water, add lime zest and all the seasonings and spices, stir until mixed, and then bring the mixture to a boil.
3. Then switch heat to medium-low level and simmer quinoa for 10 to 12 minutes until tender. When done, let the quinoa cool for 10 minutes, fluff it with a fork and transfer into a medium bowl.
4. Add rice and tomato dressing, stir until well mixed, add cherries and then toss until mixed.

Storage instructions:

Cool the rice, divide evenly between two containers, cover with a lid, and then store the containers in the refrigerator for up to 7 days.

Reheating instructions:

When ready to eat, reheat in the oven for 1 to 2 minutes until hot and then serve.

Day 6
Breakfast – Blueberry-Pie Smoothie

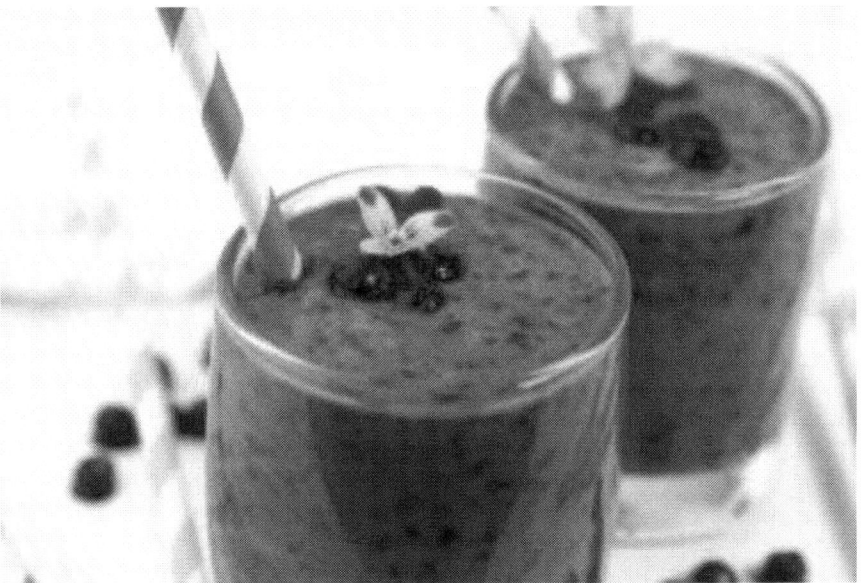

Serving: 2

Preparation time: 5 minutes; Cooking time: 0 minutes;
Nutritional Info: 302 Cal; 3 g Fats; 11 g Protein; 60 g Carb; 7 g Fiber;

Ingredients

- ¼ cup cooked amaranth
- 1 cup blueberries
- 1 teaspoon Bromide Plus Powder
- 1 burro banana, peeled
- 1 tablespoon walnut butter, homemade

Extra:

- 2 tablespoons date sugar
- 2 cups soft-jelly coconut milk, homemade
-

Directions

1. Plug in a high-speed food processor or blender and add all the ingredients in its jar.
2. Cover the blender jar with its lid and then pulse for 40 to 60 seconds until smooth.
3. Divide the drink between two glasses.

Storage instructions:

Divide drink between two jars, cover with a lid and then store the containers in the refrigerator for up to 3 days.

Lunch – Chickpea Nuggets

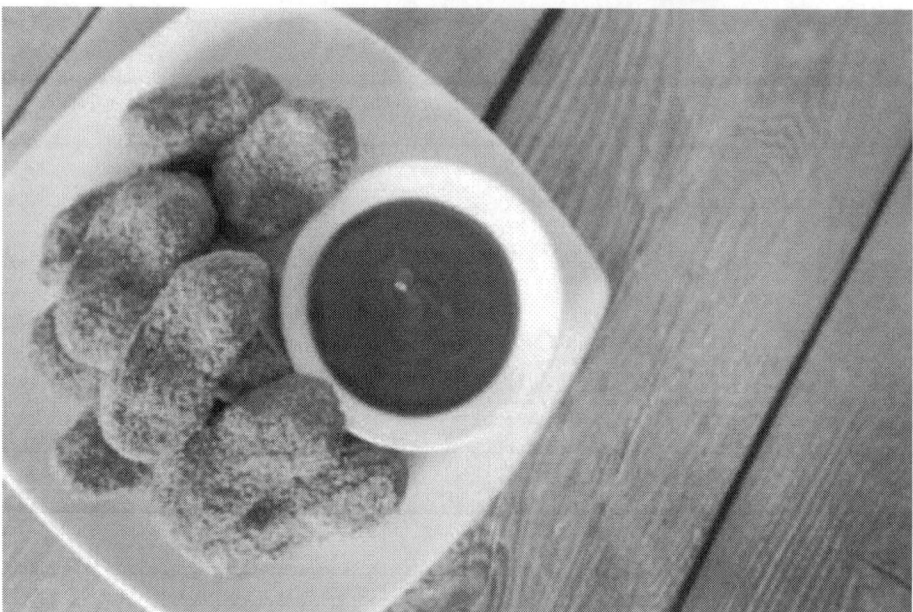

Serving: 2

Preparation time: 10 minutes; Cooking time: 30 minutes;
Nutritional Info: 291.6 Cal; 3.9 g Fats; 19.9 g Protein; 26.8 g Carb; 3.4 g Fiber;

Ingredients

- 2 cups cooked chickpeas
- ½ teaspoon salt
- 1 teaspoon onion powder
- 1/3 cup and 1 tablespoon bread crumbs

Directions

1. Switch on the oven, then set it to 350 degrees F and let it preheat.
2. Meanwhile, place chickpeas in a food processor and then pulse until crumbled.
3. Tip the chickpeas in a bowl, add remaining ingredients in it except for 1/3 cup of breadcrumbs and then stir until a chunky mixture comes together.
4. Shape the mixture into evenly sized balls, shape each ball into the nugget, arrange on a baking sheet greased with oil and then bake for 15 minutes per side until golden brown.

Storage instructions:

Cool the nuggets, divide evenly between two containers, cover with a lid, and then store the containers in the refrigerator for up to 7 days.

Reheating instructions:

When ready to eat, reheat in the oven for 1 to 2 minutes until hot and then serve.

Dinner – Squash & Apple Burger

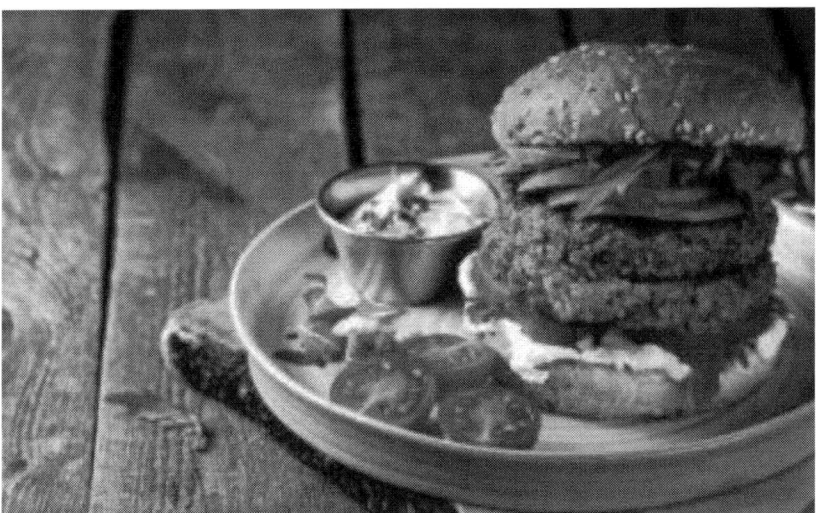

Serving: 2; **Preparation time: 10 minutes; Cooking time: 1 hour;**

Nutritional Info: 250 Cal; 4 g Fats; 6 g Protein; 51 g Carb; 5 g Fiber;

Ingredients

- ¾ cup diced butternut squash
- ½ cup diced apples
- 1 cup cooked wild rice
- ¼ cup chopped shallots
- ½ tablespoon thyme; ¼ teaspoon sea salt, divided
- 1 tablespoon pumpkin seeds, unsalted
- 1 tablespoon grapeseed oil
- 2 spelt burgers, halved, toasted

Directions

1. Switch on the oven, then set it to 400 degrees F and let it preheat.
2. Meanwhile, take a cookie sheet, line it with parchment sheet, spread squash pieces on it and then sprinkle with 1/8 teaspoon salt. Bake the squash for 15 minutes, then add shallots and apple, sprinkle with remaining salt, and then bake for 20 to 30 minutes until cooked. When done, let the vegetable mixture cool for 15 minutes, transfer it into a food processor, add thyme and then pulse until a chunky mixture comes together.
3. Add pumpkin seeds and cooked wild rice, pulse until combined, and then tip the mixture in a bowl. Taste the mixture to adjust and then shape it into two patties.
4. Take a skillet pan, place it over medium heat, add oil and when hot, place patties in it and then cook for 5 to 7 minutes per side until browned. Sandwich patties in burger.

Storage instructions:

Cool the patties, divide evenly between two containers, cover with a lid, and then store the containers in the refrigerator for up to 7 days.

Reheating instructions:

When ready to eat, reheat in the oven for 1 to 2 minutes until hot, sandwich patties in burger buns and then serve.

Day 7
Breakfast – Cucumber and Basil Cleansing Drink

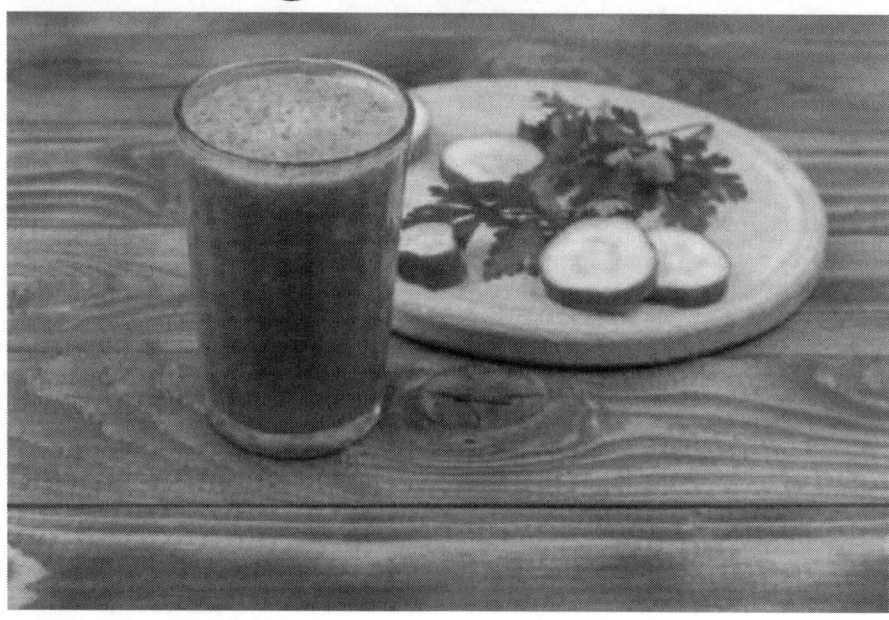

Serving: 2

Preparation time: 5 minutes; Cooking time: 0 minutes;
Nutritional Info: 56.1 Cal; 0.5 g Fats; 0.9 g Protein; 12 g Carb; 2 g Fiber;

Ingredients

- 4 cucumbers, deseeded
- 1 bunch of basil leaves
- 2 key limes, juiced
- ½ teaspoon Bromide Plus Powder
- 2 cups soft-jelly coconut water

Directions

1. Plug in a high-speed food processor or blender and add all the ingredients in its jar.
2. Cover the blender jar with its lid and then pulse for 40 to 60 seconds until smooth.
3. Divide the drink between two glasses.

Storage instructions:

Divide drink between two jars, cover with a lid and then store the containers in the refrigerator for up to 3 days.

Lunch – Banana, Pear and Coconut Smoothie

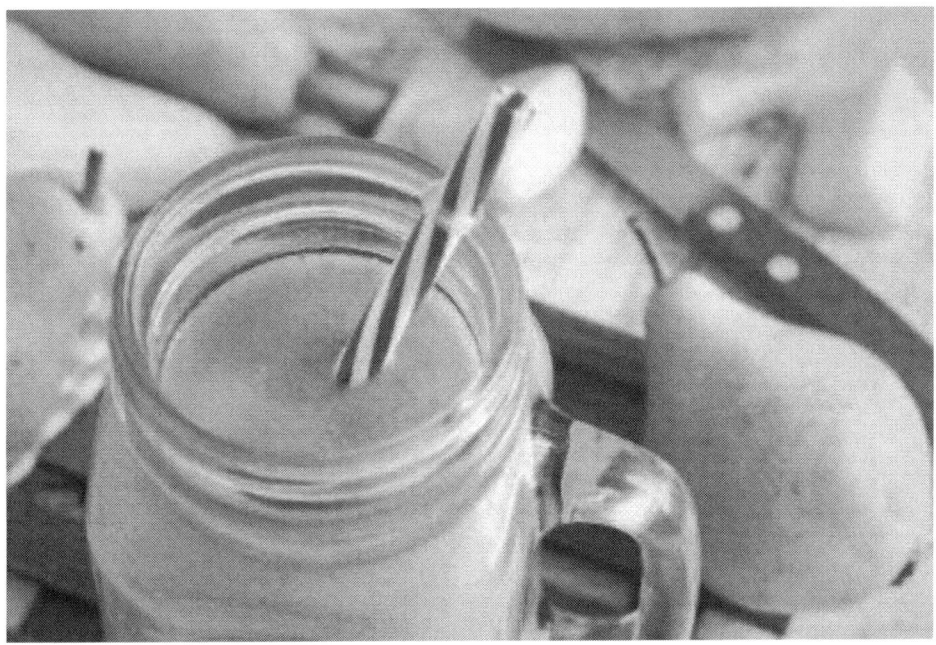

Serving: 2

Preparation time: 5 minutes; Cooking time: 0 minutes;
Nutritional Info: 90 Cal; 0 g Fats; 1 g Protein; 24 g Carb; 3 g Fiber;

Ingredients

- 1 burro banana, peeled
- 2 cups chopped kale
- 1 pear, diced
- 1 cup of soft-jelly coconut water

Directions

1. Plug in a high-speed food processor or blender and add all the ingredients in its jar.
2. Cover the blender jar with its lid and then pulse for 40 to 60 seconds until smooth.
3. Divide the drink between two glasses.

Storage instructions:

Divide drink between two jars, cover with a lid and then store the containers in the refrigerator for up to 3 days.

Dinner – Pasta with Chickpea Sauce

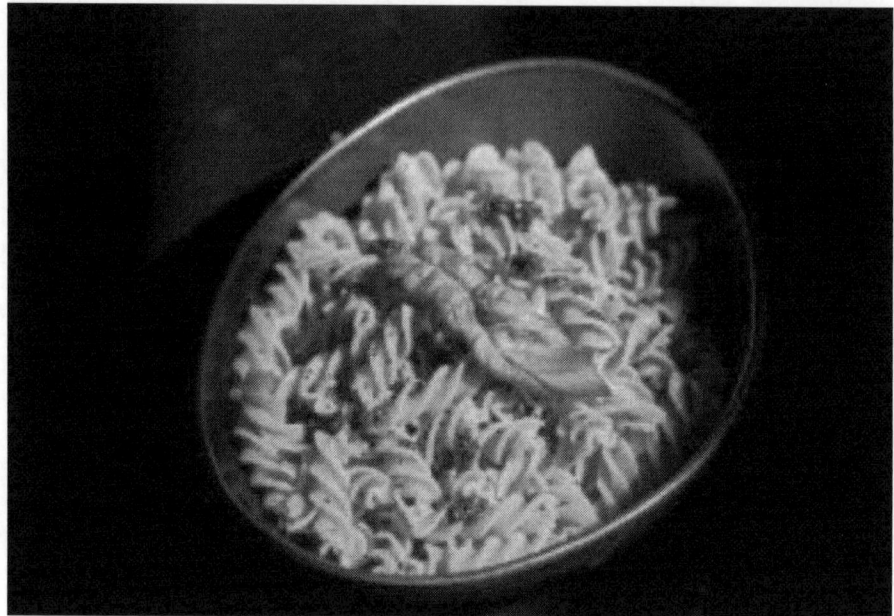

Serving: 2; **Preparation time: 10 minutes; Cooking time: 10 minutes;**

Nutritional Info: 197 Cal; 6.1 g Fats; 6 g Protein; 30.5 g Carb; 5 g Fiber;

Ingredients

- ½ cup cooked chickpeas
- 2 cups cooked spelt pasta, hot
- ½ cup chopped onion
- ½ teaspoon habanero
- 2 tablespoons chopped basil
- 1 ½ tablespoon olive oil
- 1/3 cup spring water
- ½ teaspoon salt
- ¼ teaspoon cayenne pepper
- 2 tablespoons chopped parsley

Directions

1. Take a medium skillet pan, place it over medium heat, add oil and when hot, add onion and habanero, and cook for 5 to 8 minutes until golden brown.
2. Spoon the onion mixture into a food processor, add chickpeas, salt, cayenne pepper, and water and then pulse until smooth.
3. Place pasta into a large bowl, add blended chickpea sauce, toss until mixed, and then garnish with basil and parsley.

Storage instructions:

Cool the pasta, divide evenly between two containers, cover with a lid, and then store the containers in the refrigerator for up to 7 days.

Reheating instructions:

When ready to eat, reheat in the oven for 1 to 2 minutes until hot and then serve.

Week 4
Shopping List

Shop for the following

- Sea Salt
- Minced / powdered garlic
- Grated / powdered ginger
- Cayenne pepper
- Onion powder
- Agave syrup
- Date sugar
- Spicemix
- Oregano
- Parsley
- Oregano
- Dill
- Basil
- Walnuts
- Brazil nuts
- Raisins
- Amaranth
- Amaranth greens
- Chickpea flour
- Fonio
- Liquid smoke
- Basil
- Bromide Plus Powder
- Olive oil
- Grapeseed oil
- Sesame oil
- Soft-jelly coconut water
- Homemade walnut milk
- Homemade hemp milk

- Spring water
- Dr. Sebi herbal tea
- Soft-jelly coconut water
- Soft-jelly coconut milk
- Alkaline tomato sauce
- Alkaline garlic sauce
- Tahini
- Sea moss gel
- Watermelon spears, 10 oz.
- Raspberries, 6 oz.
- Key lime, count
- Cucumber, large
- Chickpeas, 15.5 oz.
- Green onion, bunch
- Kale, bunch
- Onion, large
- Cherry tomatoes, 1 pint
- Avocado, large
- Zucchini
- Papaya, 1 lb.
- Quinoa, 16 oz.
- Button mushrooms, 8 oz.
- Wild rice, 16 oz.
- Banana
- Spelt flour, 680 g
- Sliced mushrooms, 8 oz.
- Green bell pepper, large
- Orange
- Okra, 12 oz.

Day 1
Breakfast – Watermelon and Raspberries Smoothie

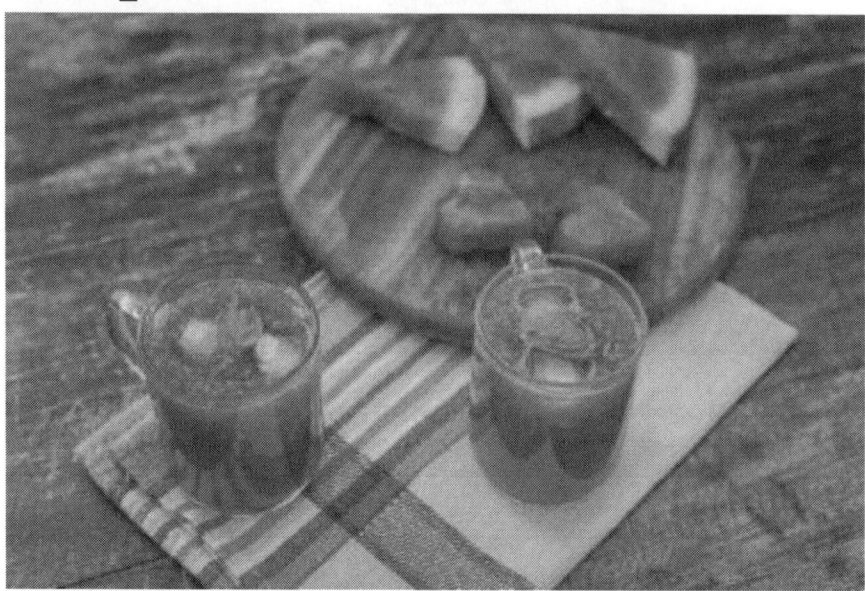

Serving: 2

Preparation time: 5 minutes; Cooking time: 0 minutes;
Nutritional Info: 110 Cal; 1 g Fats; 3.4 g Protein; 26 g Carb; 7 g Fiber;

Ingredients

- 1 cup watermelon chunks
- ½ cup raspberries
- 1 key lime, juiced
- ¼ cup cucumber, deseeded, diced
- ½ cup soft-jelly coconut water

Directions

1. Plug in a high-speed food processor or blender and add all the ingredients in its jar.
2. Cover the blender jar with its lid and then pulse for 40 to 60 seconds until smooth.
3. Divide the drink between two glasses.

Storage instructions:

Divide drink between two jars, cover with a lid and then store the containers in the refrigerator for up to 3 days.

Lunch – Mashed Potatoes

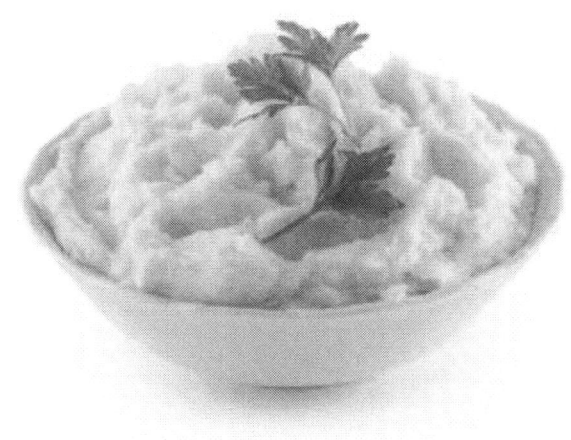

Serving: 2

Preparation time: 5 minutes; Cooking time: 10 minutes;
Nutritional Info: 52 Cal; 2.6 g Fats; 1.4 g Protein; 6 g Carb; 1.2 g Fiber;

Ingredients

- 2 cups cooked chickpeas
- 2 teaspoons onion powder
- 2 teaspoons sea salt
- ¼ cup diced green onion
- 1 cup walnut milk, homemade

Directions

1. Place chickpeas in a food processor, pour in the milk, and then pulse for 1 to 2 minutes until blended.
2. Tip the chickpea mixture into a medium saucepan, place it over medium heat, add green onions and then stir until mixed.
3. Cook the chickpeas for 25 to 30 minutes until cooked, stirring constantly.

Storage instructions:

Cool the mashed potatoes, divide evenly between two containers, cover with a lid, and then store the containers in the refrigerator for up to 7 days.

Reheating instructions:

When ready to eat, reheat in the oven for 1 to 2 minutes until hot and then serve.

Dinner – Kale and Avocado Salad

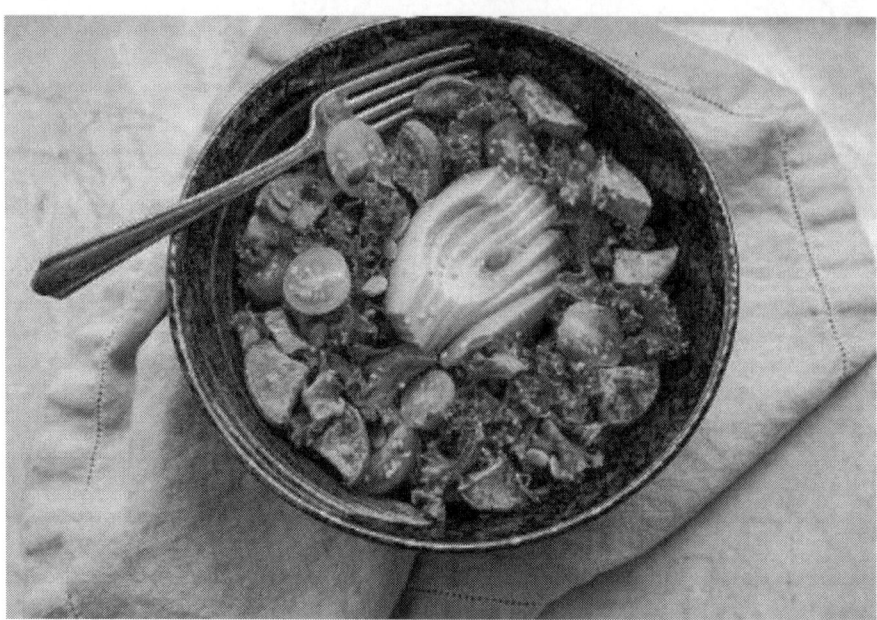

Serving: 2

Preparation time: 5 minutes; Cooking time: 0 minutes;
Nutritional Info: 143 Cal; 10.5 g Fats; 3 g Protein; 12.4 g Carb; 4.8 g Fiber;

Ingredients

- 1 bundle of kale, cut into thin strips
- 1 small white onion, peeled, chopped
- 12 cherry tomatoes, chopped
- 1 tablespoon salt
- 1 avocado, peeled, pitted, sliced

Directions

1. Take a large bowl, place kale strips in it, sprinkle with salt, and then massage for 2 minutes.
2. Cover the bowl with a plastic wrap or its lid, let it rest for a minimum of 30 minutes, and then stir in onion and tomatoes until well combined.
3. Let the salad sit for 5 minutes, add avocado slices.

Storage instructions:

Divide the salad without avocado evenly between two containers, cover with a lid, and then store the containers in the refrigerator for up to 5 days.

Reheating instructions:

When ready to eat, add avocado slices in it and then serve.

Day 2
Breakfast – Zucchini Bacon

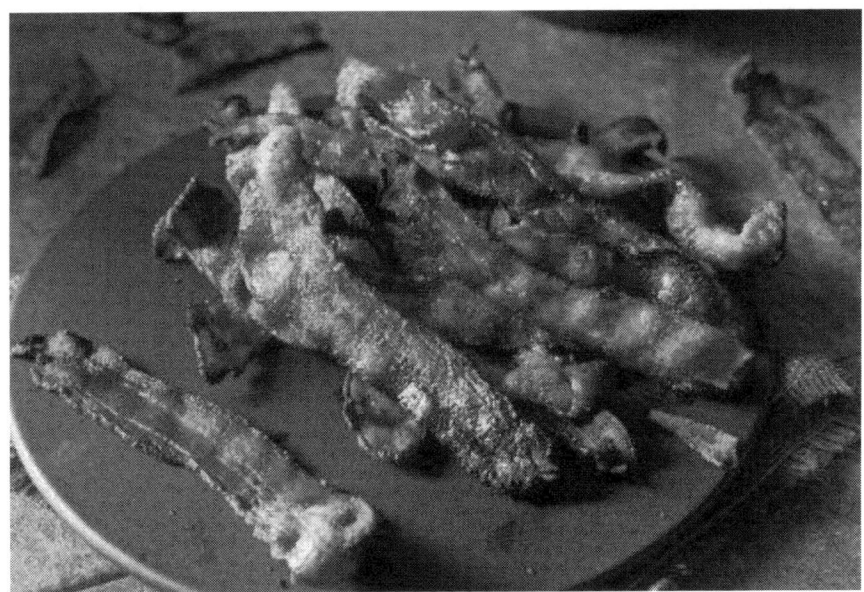

Serving: 2; **Preparation time: 10 minutes; Cooking time: 20 minutes;**

Nutritional Info: 184 Cal; 2 g Fats; 12 g Protein; 26 g Carb; 2 g Fiber;

Ingredients

- 2 zucchini, cut into strips
- 1 tablespoon onion powder
- ½ teaspoon ginger powder
- 1 tablespoon of sea salt; ½ teaspoon cayenne powder
- ¼ cup date sugar; 2 tablespoons agave syrup
- 1 teaspoon liquid smoke; ¼ cup spring water
- 1 tablespoon grapeseed oil

Directions

1. Take a medium saucepan, place it over medium heat, add all the ingredients except for zucchini and oil and then cook until sugar has dissolved.
2. Then place zucchini strips in a large bowl, pour in the mixture from the saucepan, toss until coated, and then let it marinate for a minimum of 1 hour.
3. When ready to cook, switch on the oven, set it to 400 degrees F, and let it preheat.
4. Take a baking sheet, line it with parchment sheet, grease with oil, arrange marinated zucchini strips on it, and then bake for 10 minutes.
5. Then flip the zucchini, continue cooking for 4 minutes and then let cool completely.

Storage instructions:

Cool the bacon, divide evenly between two containers, cover with a lid, and then store the containers in the refrigerator for up to 7 days.

Reheating instructions:

When ready to eat, reheat in the oven for 1 to 2 minutes until hot and then serve.

Lunch – Papaya and Quinoa Smoothie

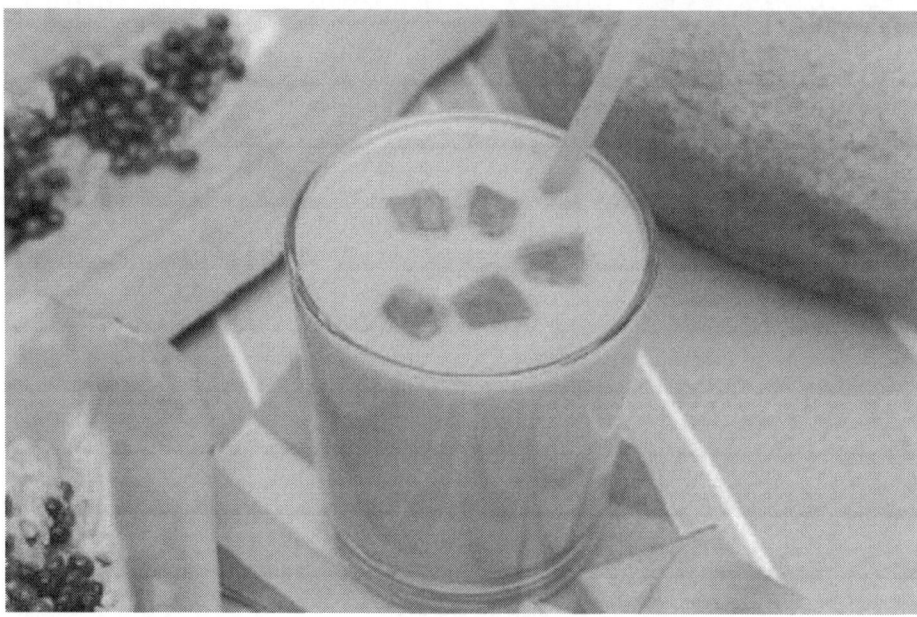

Serving: 2

Preparation time: 5 minutes; Cooking time: 10 minutes;
Nutritional Info: 224.6 Cal; 7.7 g Fats; 7 g Protein; 33.7 g Carb; 3.5 g Fiber;

Ingredients

- 2 cups papaya cubes
- 2 tablespoons date sugar
- 1 cup cooked quinoa or amaranth
- 2 teaspoons Bromide Plus Powder
- 2 cups hemp milk, homemade

Directions

1. Plug in a high-speed food processor or blender and add all the ingredients in its jar.
2. Cover the blender jar with its lid and then pulse for 40 to 60 seconds until smooth.
3. Divide the drink between two glasses.

Storage instructions:

Divide drink between two jars, cover with a lid and then store the containers in the refrigerator for up to 3 days.

Dinner – Mushroom and Kale Stir-fry with Wild Rice

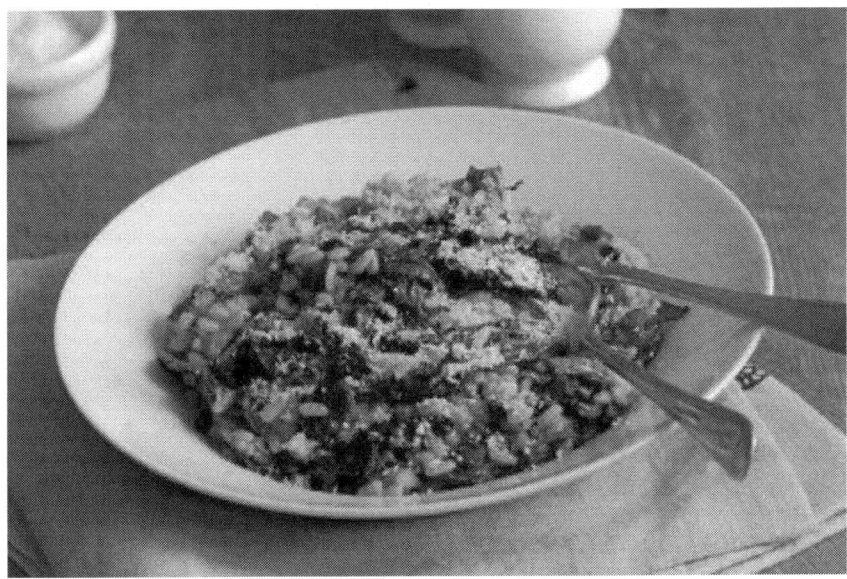

Serving: 2

Preparation time: 5 minutes; Cooking time: 15 minutes;
Nutritional Info: 234 Cal; 13 g Fats; 6 g Protein; 22 g Carb; 6 g Fiber;

Ingredients

- ½ of medium white onion, peeled, diced
- 10 button mushrooms, sliced
- 1 cup Kale leaves
- 2 cups cooked wild rice

Extra:

- 1 tablespoon grapeseed oil
- 2/3 teaspoon salt
- ¼ teaspoon cayenne pepper

Directions

1. Take a large skillet pan, place it over medium heat, add oil and when hot, add onion, and then cook for 4 minutes until tender.
2. Add mushrooms, stir until mixed and cook for 4 minutes until mushrooms have almost tender.
3. Add wild rice and kale into the pan, season with salt and cayenne pepper, stir until mixed, and then cook for 5 minutes until kale leaves wilts.

Storage instructions:

Cool the rice, divide evenly between two containers, cover with a lid, and then store the containers in the refrigerator for up to 7 days.

Reheating instructions:

When ready to eat, reheat in the oven for 1 to 2 minutes until hot and then serve.

Day 3
Breakfast – Spelt Banana Bread

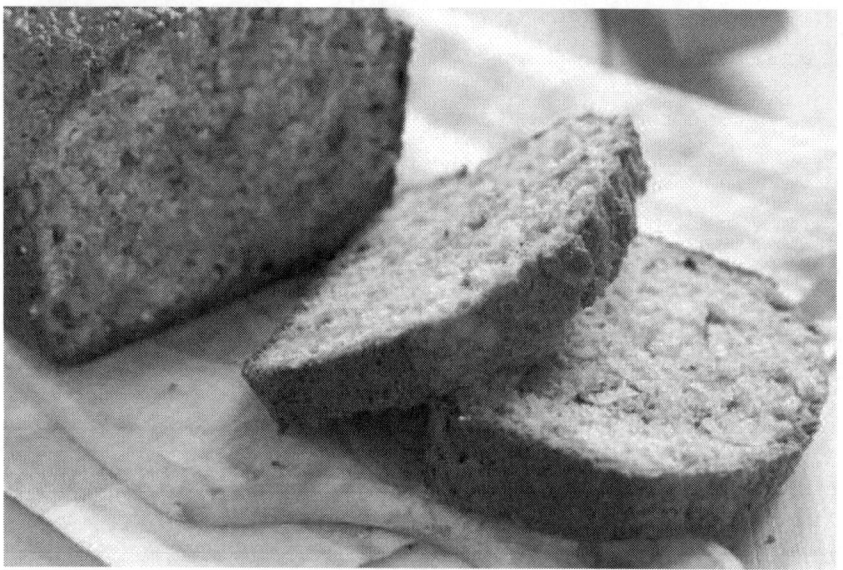

Serving: 2; Preparation time: 10 minutes; Cooking time: 20 minutes;

Nutritional Info: 186 Cal; 11.3 g Fats; 1.3 g Protein; 22 g Carb; 2 g Fiber;

Ingredients

- 1/3 cup chopped walnuts
- 1 1/3 cup of burro banana
- 2/3 cup spelt flour
- 1/8 teaspoon salt
- ¼ cup agave syrup
- 1 1/3 tablespoons olive oil

Directions

1. Switch on the oven, then set it to 350 degrees F and let it preheat.
2. Meanwhile, place the banana in a medium bowl, mash it by using a fork and then stir in oil and agave syrup until combined.
3. Take a separate medium bowl, place flour in it, add salt and nuts, stir until mixed, and then stir in the banana mixture until smooth.
4. Pour the batter into a parchment-lined loaf pan and then bake for 20 minutes until firm and the top turn golden brown.
5. When done, let the bread cool for 10 minutes, then cut it into slices.

Storage instructions:

Cover each bread slice in a plastic wrap and foil and then store in the refrigerator for up to 7 days.

Reheating instructions:

When ready to eat, bring the bread slices to room temperature or reheat in the oven for 1 to 2 minutes until warm and then serve.

Lunch – Veggie Fritters

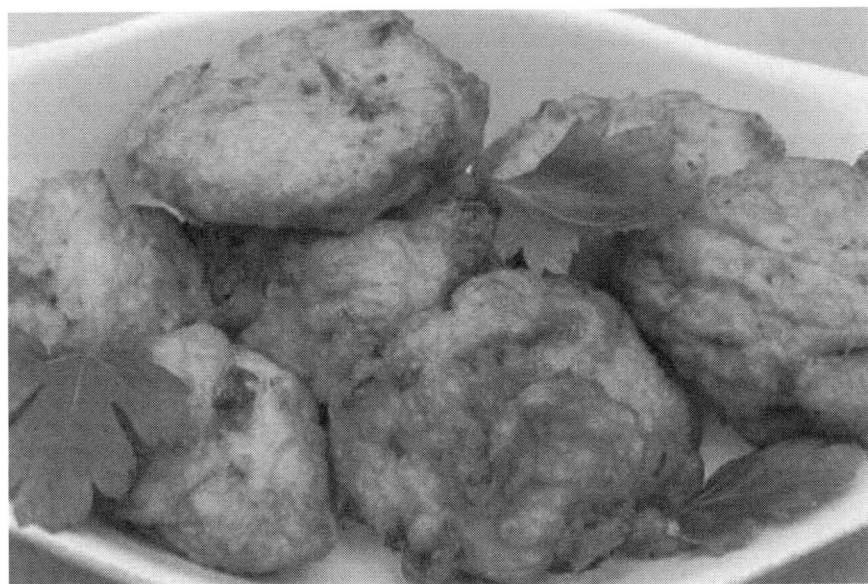

Serving: 2; **Preparation time: 10 minutes; Cooking time: 10 minutes;**

Nutritional Info: 281.5 Cal; 15.2 g Fats; 13.8 g Protein; 26.2 g Carb; 5 g Fiber;

Ingredients

- 1 cup chickpea flour
- 200g mushrooms, chopped
- 1 medium green bell pepper, cored, chopped
- 1 tablespoon onion powder
- 2 medium white onions, peeled, chopped

Extra:

- 1 teaspoon of sea salt; 1 tablespoon oregano
- 1/8 teaspoon cayenne pepper; 1 tablespoon grapeseed oil
- 1 tablespoon basil leaves, chopped
- ½ cup spring water

Directions

1. Take a large bowl, place all the vegetables in it, add all the seasonings, basil and oregano, stir until mixed, and then let the mixture rest for 5 minutes.
2. Add chickpea flour, stir until mixed and then stir in water until well combined and smooth.
3. Take a large skillet, and place over medium heat, add oil and when hot, ladle vegetable mixture in it in portions, press down each portion, and then cook for 3 to 4 minutes per side until cooked and golden brown.

Storage instructions:

Cool the fritters, divide evenly between two containers, cover with a lid, and then store the containers in the refrigerator for up to 7 days.

Reheating instructions:

When ready to eat, reheat in the oven for 1 to 2 minutes until hot and then serve.

Dinner – Chickpea and Mushroom Curry

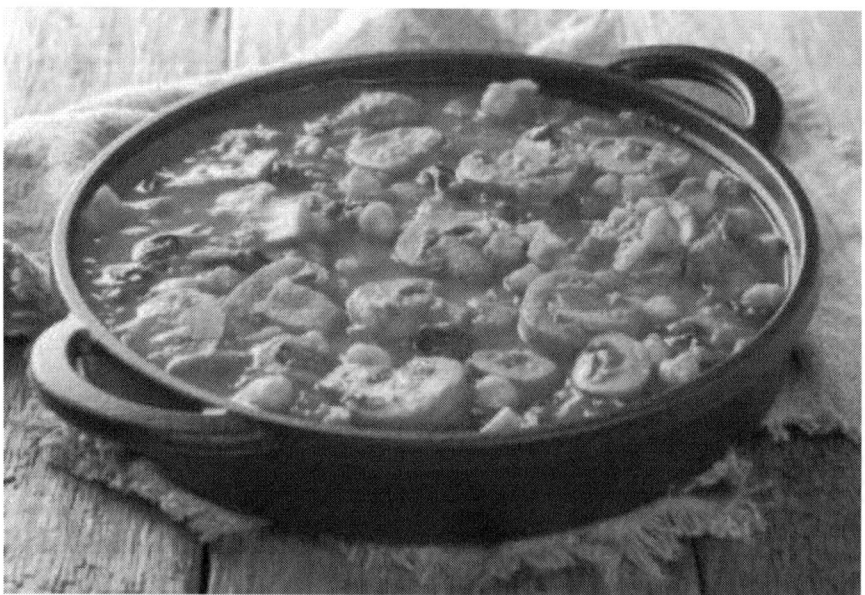

Serving: 2

Preparation time: 5 minutes; Cooking time: 12 minutes;
Nutritional Info: 194.7 Cal; 8.5 g Fats; 5.8 g Protein; 25.7 g Carb; 5.4 g Fiber;

Ingredients

- 1 cup cooked chickpea
- 1 small white onion, peeled, diced
- ½ of medium green bell pepper, cored, chopped
- 1 cup diced mushrooms
- 8 cherry tomatoes, chopped

Extra:

- ½ teaspoon salt
- ¼ teaspoon cayenne pepper
- 1 teaspoon grapeseed oil

Directions

1. Take a medium skillet, and place over medium heat, add oil and when hot, add onion, tomatoes, and bell pepper and then cook for 2 minutes.
2. Add chickpeas and mushrooms, season with and cayenne pepper, stir until combined, and switch heat to medium-low level and then simmer for 10 minutes until cooked, covering the pan with its lid.

Storage instructions:

Cool the curry, divide evenly between two containers, cover with a lid, and then store the containers in the refrigerator for up to 7 days.

Reheating instructions:

When ready to eat, reheat in the oven for 1 to 2 minutes until hot and then serve.

Day 4
Breakfast – Avocado and Cucumber Smoothie

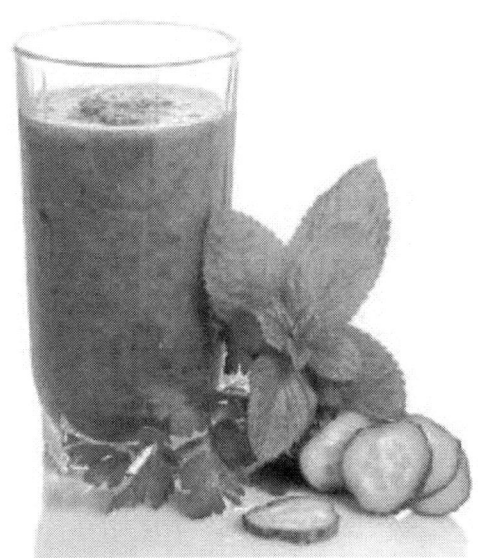

Serving: 2

Preparation time: 5 minutes; Cooking time: 0 minutes;
Nutritional Info: 103 Cal; 4.5 g Fats; 1.6 g Protein; 16.2 g Carb; 2.5 g Fiber;

Ingredients

- 1 burro banana, peeled
- ¼ of an avocado
- ¼ of a cucumber
- 1 tablespoon agave syrup
- ½ cup herbal tea

Extra:

- 1 tablespoon chopped walnuts
- 1 cup soft-jelly coconut milk, homemade

Directions

1. Plug in a high-speed food processor or blender and add all the ingredients in its jar.
2. Cover the blender jar with its lid and then pulse for 40 to 60 seconds until smooth.
3. Divide the drink between two glasses.

Storage instructions:

Divide drink between two jars, cover with a lid and then store the containers in the refrigerator for up to 3 days.

Lunch – Fonio Salad

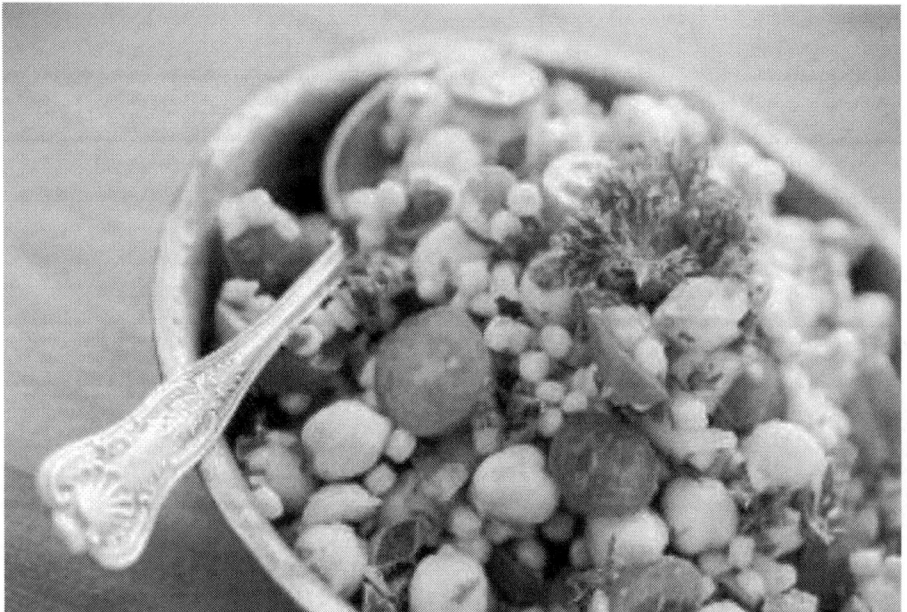

Serving: 2; **Preparation time: 10 minutes; Cooking time: 5 minutes;**

Nutritional Info: 145 Cal; 3 g Fats; 6 g Protein; 24.5 g Carb; 5.5 g Fiber;

Ingredients

- ½ cup cooked chickpeas
- ¼ cup chopped cucumber
- ½ cup chopped red pepper
- ½ cup cherry tomatoes, halved
- ½ cup fonio

Extra:

- 1/3 teaspoon salt
- 1 tablespoon grapeseed oil
- 1/8 teaspoon cayenne pepper
- 1 key lime, juiced
- 2 tablespoon chopped parsley
- 1 cup spring water

Directions

1. Take a medium saucepan, place it over high heat, pour in water, and bring it to boil.
2. Add fonio, switch heat to the low level, cook for 1 minute, and then remove the pan from heat. Cover the pan with its lid, let fonio rest for 5 minutes, fluff by using a fork and then let it cool for 15 minutes.
3. Take a salad bowl, place lime juice and oil in it and then stir in salt and cayenne pepper until combined. Add remaining ingredients including fonio, toss until mixed.

Storage instructions:

Divide the salad evenly between two containers, cover with a lid, and then store the containers in the refrigerator for up to 5 days.

Dinner – Vegetable Low Mein

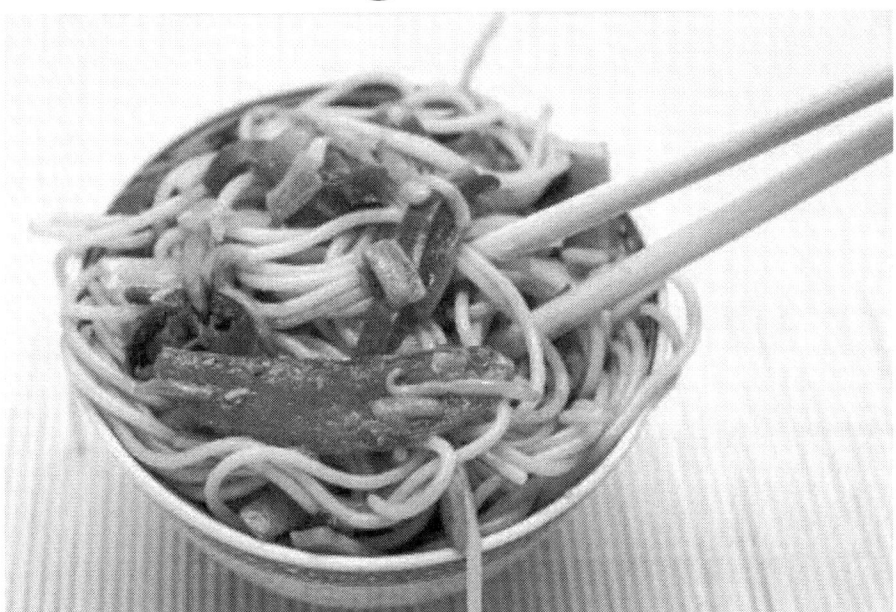

Serving: 2

Preparation time: 5 minutes; Cooking time: 10 minutes;
Nutritional Info: 330 Cal; 11 g Fats; 10 g Protein; 48 g Carb; 4 g Fiber;

Ingredients

- 2 cups cooked spelt noodles
- ½ of medium green bell pepper, cored, sliced
- ½ of medium red bell pepper, cored, sliced
- 1 medium white onion, cored, sliced
- ½ cup sliced mushrooms

Extra:

- 2/3 teaspoon salt
- ¼ teaspoon onion powder
- 1/3 teaspoon cayenne pepper
- 1 key lime juiced
- 1 tablespoon sesame oil

Directions

1. Take a large skillet pan, place it over medium heat, add oil and when hot, add all the vegetables and cook for 3 to 5 minutes until tender-crisp.
2. Add all the spices, drizzle with lime juice, stir until mixed, and then cook for 1 minute.
3. Add noodles, toss until well mixed and then cook for 2 to 3 minutes until hot.

Storage instructions:

Cool the noodles, divide evenly between two containers, cover with a lid, and then store the containers in the refrigerator for up to 7 days.

Reheating instructions:

When ready to eat, reheat in the oven for 1 to 2 minutes until hot and then serve.

Day 5
Breakfast – Orange and Banana Drink

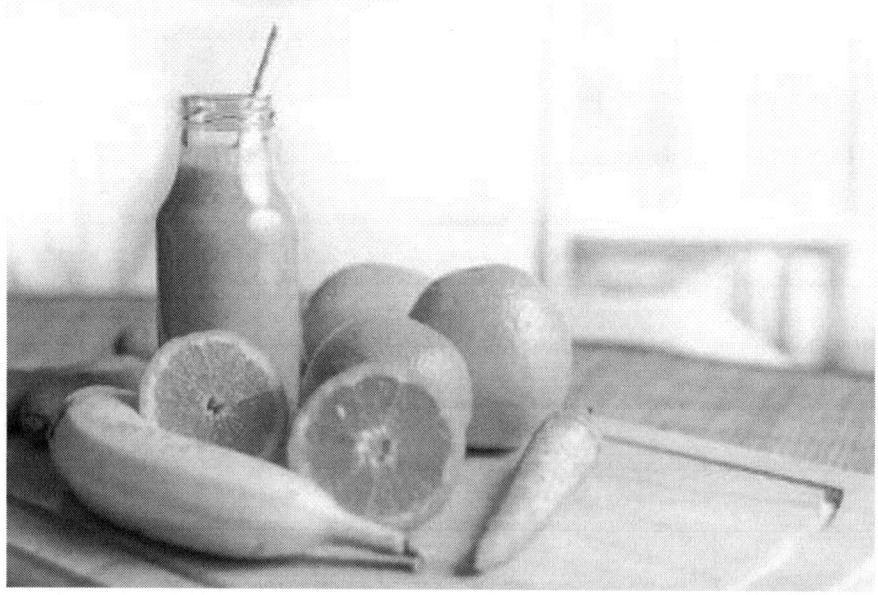

Serving: 2

Preparation time: 5 minutes; Cooking time: 0 minutes;
Nutritional Info: 138.5 Cal; 0.6 g Fats; 1.5 g Protein; 35.1 g Carb; 4.7 g Fiber;

Ingredients

- ½ of a burro banana, peeled
- 3 oranges, peeled
- 1 ½ tablespoons Date sugar
- ½ teaspoon Bromide Plus Powder
- 1 cup of soft-jelly coconut water

Directions

1. Plug in a high-speed food processor or blender and add all the ingredients in its jar.
2. Cover the blender jar with its lid and then pulse for 40 to 60 seconds until smooth.
3. Divide the drink between two glasses.

Storage instructions:

Divide drink between two jars, cover with a lid and then store the containers in the refrigerator for up to 3 days.

Lunch – Blueberry Spelt Pancakes

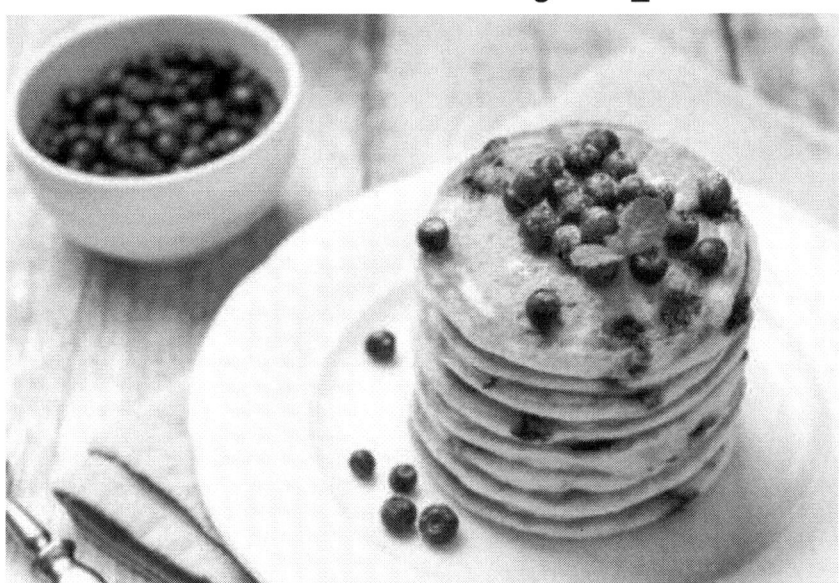

Serving: 2

Preparation time: 10 minutes; Cooking time: 8 minutes;
Nutritional Info: 156 Cal; 3.6 g Fats; 8.4 g Protein; 22.8 g Carb; 3.3 g Fiber;

Ingredients

- 1 cup spelt flour
- ¼ cup blueberries
- ¼ cup agave syrup
- 1/8 teaspoon sea moss
- ½ cup soft-jelly coconut milk

Extra:

- ¼ cup spring water
- 2 tablespoons grapeseed oil

Directions

1. Take a large bowl, place flour in it, add agave syrup, 1 tablespoon oil and sea moss, and then stir until mixed.
2. Whisk in milk and water until smooth batter comes together and then fold in berries.
3. Take a large skillet pan, place it over medium heat, add remaining oil and when hot, ladle batter in it, shape into a pancake and then cook for 2 to 3 minutes per side until golden brown and cooked.

Storage instructions:

Cool the pancakes, divide evenly between two containers, cover with a lid, and then store the containers in the refrigerator for up to 7 days.

Reheating instructions:

When ready to eat, reheat in the oven for 1 to 2 minutes until hot and then serve.

Dinner – Spiced Okra Curry

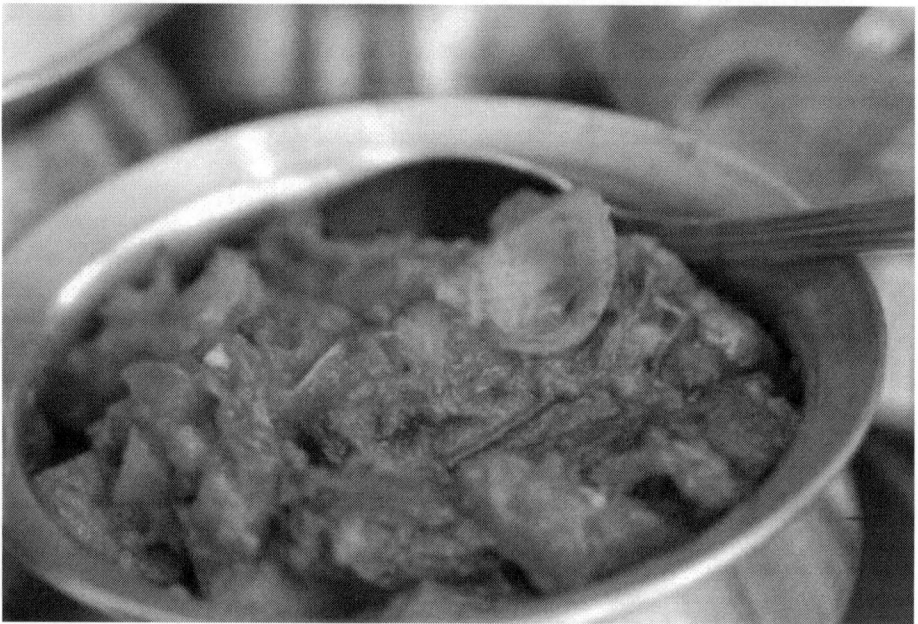

Serving: 2; **Preparation time: 5 minutes; Cooking time: 10 minutes;**

Nutritional Info: 137 Cal; 8.4 g Fats; 4 g Protein; 15 g Carb; 5.6 g Fiber;

Ingredients

- 1 ½ cup okra
- 8 cherry tomatoes, chopped
- 1 medium onion, peeled, sliced
- ¾ cup vegetable broth, homemade

Extra:

- 6 teaspoons spice mix
- ¼ teaspoon salt; ½ tablespoon grapeseed oil
- ¼ teaspoon cayenne pepper
- ¾ cup tomato sauce, alkaline
- 6 tablespoons soft-jelly coconut milk

Directions

1. Take a large skillet pan, place it over medium heat, add oil and warm, add onion, and then cook for 5 minutes until golden brown.
2. Add spice mix, add remaining ingredients into the pan except for okra, stir until mixed, and then bring the mixture to a simmer.
3. Add okra, stir until mixed, and then cook for 10 to 15 minutes over medium-low heat setting until cooked.

Storage instructions:

Cool the curry, divide evenly between two containers, cover with a lid, and then store the containers in the refrigerator for up to 7 days.

Reheating instructions:

When ready to eat, reheat in the oven for 1 to 2 minutes until hot and then serve.

Day 6
Breakfast – Lettuce, Banana and Berries Smoothie

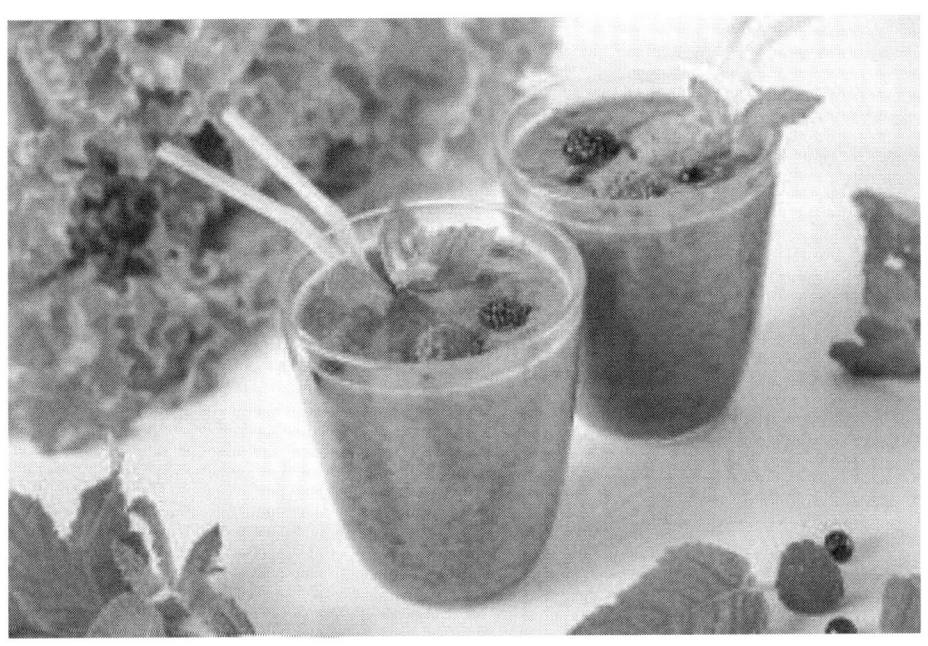

Serving: 2

Preparation time: 5 minutes; Cooking time: 0 minutes;
Nutritional Info: 147 Cal; 0.8 g Fats; 3.3 g Protein; 36 g Carb; 4 g Fiber;

Ingredients

- ½ of a burro banana
- ¼ cup blueberries
- 1 cup Romaine lettuce
- 2 tablespoons key lime juice
- ½ cup soft jelly coconut water

Extra:

- ½ cup of ginger tea

Directions

1. Plug in a high-speed food processor or blender and add all the ingredients in its jar.
2. Cover the blender jar with its lid and then pulse for 40 to 60 seconds until smooth.
3. Divide the drink between two glasses.

Storage instructions:

Divide drink between two jars, cover with a lid and then store the containers in the refrigerator for up to 3 days.

Lunch – Falafel

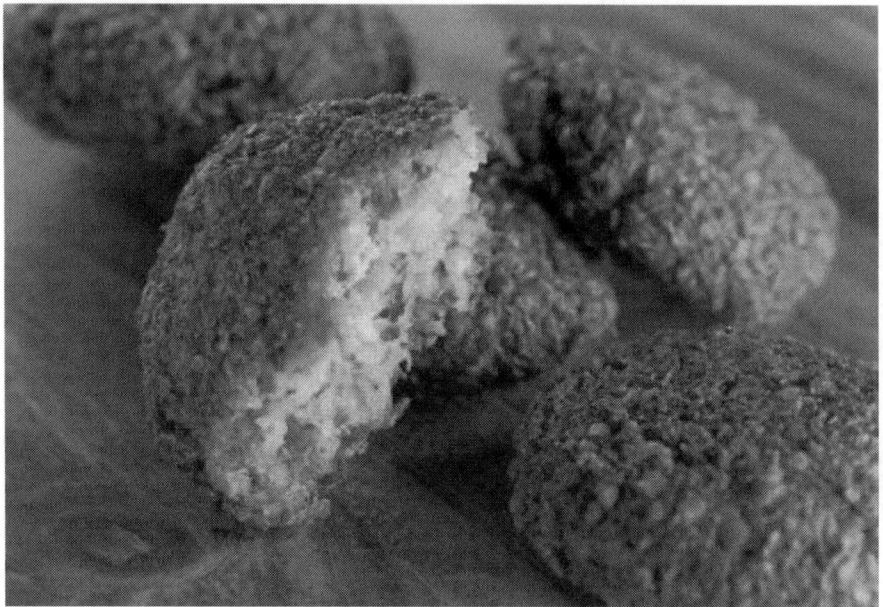

Serving: 2; **Preparation time: 10 minutes; Cooking time: 10 minutes;**

Nutritional Info: 182 Cal; 10 g Fats; 6 g Protein; 18 g Carb; 4 g Fiber;

Ingredients

- 2 cups cooked chickpeas
- ½ cup chopped white onion
- ½ cup chickpea flour
- ¼ cup green onions, chopped
- 1 teaspoon chopped basil

Extra:

- 1 teaspoon chopped oregano; 1 teaspoon onion powder
- ½ teaspoon of sea salt; ½ teaspoon cayenne pepper
- 1/3 cup water from cooked chickpeas
- 1 tablespoon lime juice; 2 tablespoons sauce, alkaline
- 1 tablespoon tahini; 1 tablespoon grapeseed oil

Directions

1. Add chickpeas into a food processor, add remaining ingredients except for oil and then pulse until well blended.
2. Tip the mixture into a bowl and then shape into even size patties.
3. Take a large skillet pan, place it over medium heat, add oil and when hot, place prepared falafel patties in it and then cook for 4 to 5 minutes per side until golden brown and cooked.

Storage instructions:

Cool the falafel, divide evenly between two containers, cover with a lid, and then store the containers in the refrigerator for up to 7 days.

Reheating instructions:

When ready to eat, reheat in the oven for 1 to 2 minutes until hot and then serve.

Dinner – Sloppy Joe

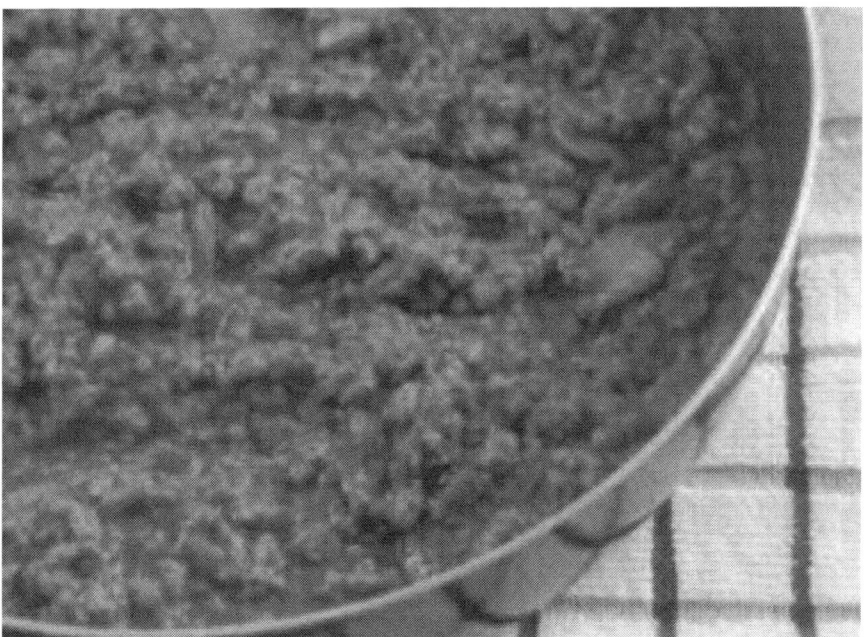

Serving: 2

Preparation time: 5 minutes; Cooking time: 12 minutes;
Nutritional Info: 166.5 Cal; 2.5 g Fats; 7 g Protein; 32.5 g Carb; 6 g Fiber;

Ingredients

- ¼ cup chopped white onion
- 1 cup cooked Kamut
- ¼ cup chopped green bell pepper
- ½ cup cooked chickpeas
- ¾ cup Barbecue Sauce, Alkaline

Extra:

- ½ teaspoon of sea salt; 1/8 teaspoon cayenne powder
- ½ teaspoon onion powder
- ½ tablespoon grapeseed oil

Directions

1. Place chickpeas and Kamut in a food processor and then pulse until combined.
2. Then take a large skillet pan, place it over medium-high heat, add oil and when hot, add onion and peppers into the pan, stir in all the seasonings and then cook for 5 minutes until tender.
3. Add blended chickpea mixture, add remaining ingredients, stir until mixed, and then simmer it for 5 minutes.

Storage instructions:

Cool the sloppy joes, divide evenly between two containers, cover with a lid, and then store the containers in the refrigerator for up to 7 days.

Reheating instructions:

When ready to eat, reheat in the oven for 1 to 2 minutes until hot and then serve.

Day 7
Breakfast – Apple, Quinoa and Fig Smoothie

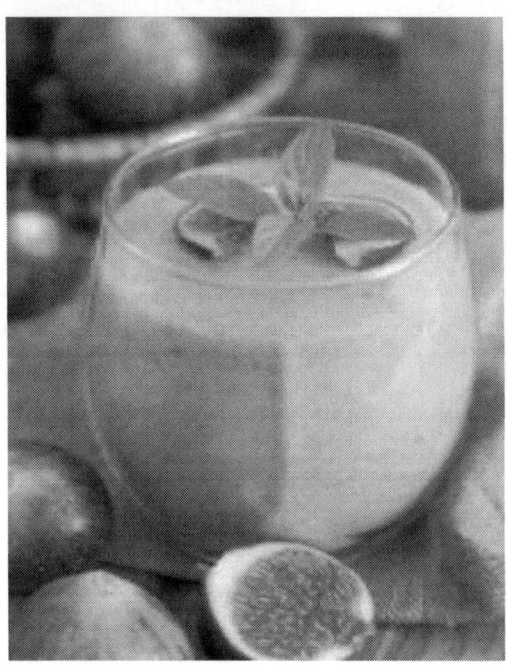

Serving: 2

Preparation time: 5 minutes; Cooking time: 0 minutes;
Nutritional Info: 153 Cal; 1 g Fats; 3 g Protein; 28 g Carb; 3 g Fiber;

Ingredients

- ½ cup cooked quinoa
- ½ of a large red apple, cored
- 1 cup amaranth greens
- 1 fig
- 1 teaspoon Bromide Plus Powder

Extra:

- 1 tablespoon raisins
- 1 tablespoon date sugar
- 1 cup hemp seed milk, homemade

Directions

1. Plug in a high-speed food processor or blender and add all the ingredients in its jar.
2. Cover the blender jar with its lid and then pulse for 40 to 60 seconds until smooth.
3. Divide the drink between two glasses.

Storage instructions:

Divide drink between two jars, cover with a lid and then store the containers in the refrigerator for up to 3 days.

Lunch – Strawberry Shake

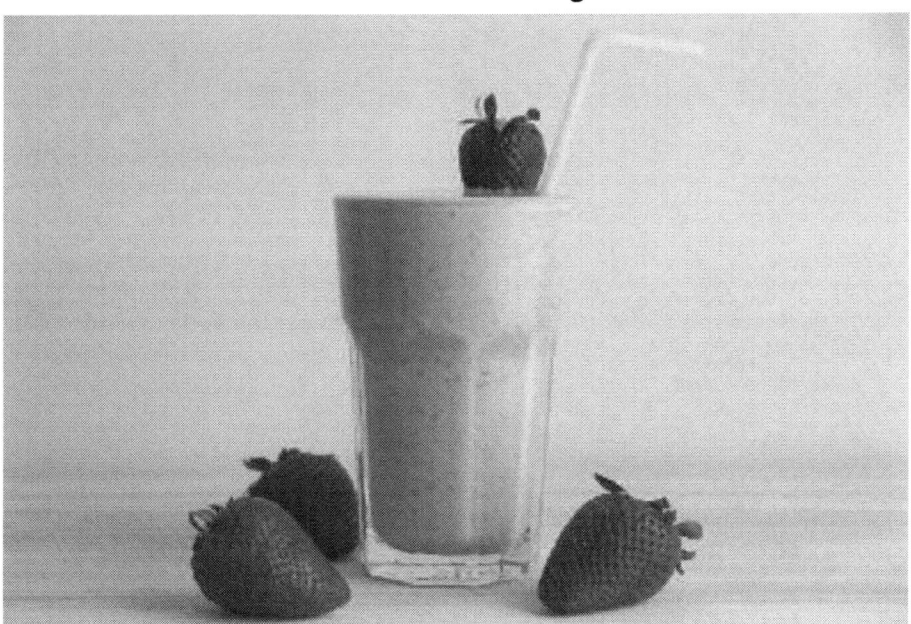

Serving: 2

Preparation time: 5 minutes; Cooking time: 10 minutes;
Nutritional Info: 137 Cal; 5 g Fats; 1 g Protein; 22 g Carb; 2 g Fiber;

Ingredients

- 1 cup strawberries
- ½ cup Brazil nuts, soaked
- 1 tablespoon agave syrup
- 1/3 cup Irish Moss gel
- 1 ½ cups spring water

Directions

1. Plug in a high-speed food processor or blender and add all the ingredients in its jar.
2. Cover the blender jar with its lid and then pulse for 40 to 60 seconds until smooth.
3. Divide the drink between two glasses.

Storage instructions:

Divide drink between two jars, cover with a lid and then store the containers in the refrigerator for up to 3 days.

Dinner – Sausage Links

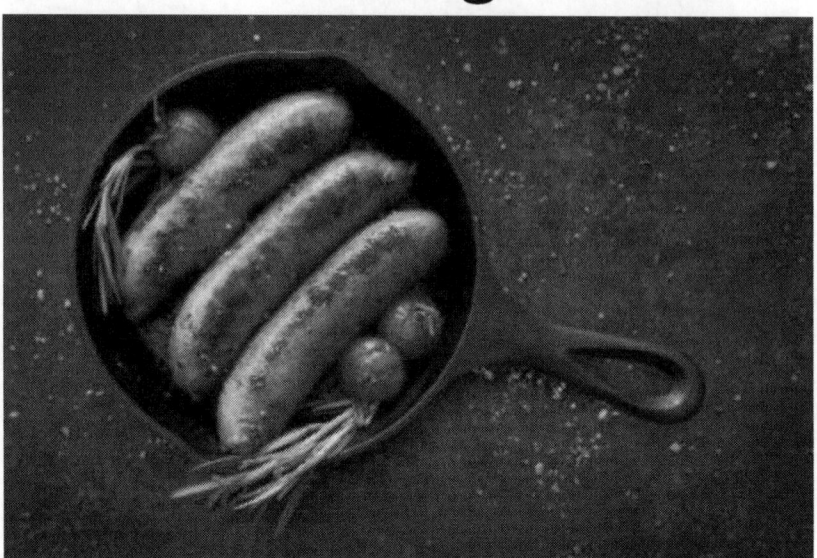

Serving: 2; **Preparation time: 10 minutes; Cooking time: 10 minutes;**

Nutritional Info: 187.1 Cal; 7.4 g Fats; 7.3 g Protein; 24.2 g Carb; 6.3 g Fiber;

Ingredients

- 1 cup cooked chickpeas
- 2 cherry tomatoes
- ½ cup sliced mushrooms
- ¼ cup chopped white onion
- ¼ cup chickpea flour

Extra:

- ½ teaspoon basil
- ½ teaspoon oregano
- ½ teaspoon of sea salt; ½ teaspoon cayenne powder
- ½ teaspoon dill
- 1 tablespoon grapeseed oil

Directions

1. Place all the ingredients in a food processor except for chickpeas and then pulse until mixed.
2. Add chickpeas, blend again until well combined, and then spoon the mixture into a piping bag.
3. Take a large pan, and place over medium-high heat, add oil and then hot, squeeze chickpea mixture to make sausage links, and then cook for 3 to 4 minutes per side until nicely brown and cooked.

Storage instructions:

Cool the sausages, divide evenly between two containers, cover with a lid, and then store the containers in the refrigerator for up to 7 days.

Reheating instructions:

When ready to eat, reheat in the oven for 1 to 2 minutes until hot and then serve.

Manufactured by Amazon.ca
Bolton, ON